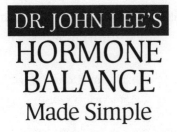

DR. JOHN LEE'S
HORMONE BALANCE
Made Simple

Also by John R. Lee, M.D., and Virginia Hopkins

What Your Doctor May Not Tell You About Menopause

What Your Doctor May Not Tell You About Premenopause

What Your Doctor May Not Tell You About Breast Cancer

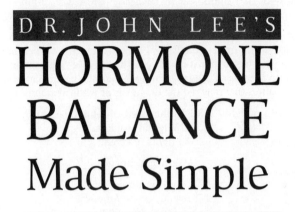

DR. JOHN LEE'S
HORMONE
BALANCE
Made Simple

**THE ESSENTIAL HOW-TO GUIDE
TO SYMPTOMS, DOSAGE, TIMING,
AND MORE**

John R. Lee, M.D.,
and
Virginia Hopkins

**WARNER
WELLNESS**

NEW YORK   BOSTON

The information herein is not intended to replace the services of trained health professionals nor be a substitute for medical advice. You are advised to consult with your health care professional with regard to matters relating to your health, and in particular regarding matters that may require diagnosis or medical attention.

Warner Wellness

Warner Books
1271 Avenue of the Americas
New York, NY 10020

Warner Wellness and the Warner Wellness logo are trademarks.

Printed in the United States of America

First Edition: August 2006

10 9 8 7 6 5 4 3 2 1

Library of Congress Cataloging-in-Publication Data

Lee, John R., M.D.
    Dr. John Lee's hormone balance made simple :
the essential how-to guide to symptoms, dosage, timing, and more / John R. Lee and Virginia Hopkins—1st ed.
        p. cm.
    Includes index.
    ISBN-13: 978-0-446-69438-4
    ISBN-10: 0-446-69438-X
    1. Hormone therapy—Popular works.   2. Menopause—Complications—Alternative treatment.   3. Premenstrual syndrome—Alternative treatment.   4. Women—Health and hygiene.   I. Hopkins, Virginia.   II. Title.
    RM286.L44 2006
    615'.36—dc22   2005023750

This book is dedicated to those doctors who love the practice of medicine so much they have the integrity to admit when something isn't working, the passion to search for a better way, and the courage to speak the truth when they find it.

Acknowledgments

Pat Lee, Dr. Lee's widow, would like to acknowledge that she and Dr. Lee's friends and colleagues will continue his work.

Virginia Hopkins would like to acknowledge the many doctors and researchers who have put their careers on the line to make bioidentical hormones available to women. Dr. David Zava has been untiring in his dedication to continuing Dr. Lee's work. It would not have been possible to complete this book without him. Helene Leonetti, M.D., and Kenna Stephenson, M.D., doggedly pursue their research projects with bioidentical hormones in spite of enormous challenges. Robert Gottesman, M.D., is a true healer and a true friend whose clinical insights have added greatly to Dr. Lee's work. C. W. Randolph, M.D., reminds us all just how rewarding a medical practice can be when it's based on a caring, informed and natural approach to women's health. Sharon MacFarland has invested time, expertise, and financial resources far beyond anyone else in the industry to fight for a woman's right to choose natural alternatives in medicine.

Contents

Contents

Foreword

This is the last project that Dr. Lee and I worked on before he died. It was possible to complete this book without his physical presence because much of the information has already been said in print, either in our books or newsletters, or on our website, not to mention in the thousands of letters and e-mails we both answered over the years. *Hormone Balance Made Simple* is the first time all of this information will be compiled into one source. It is just what the cover implies—a simple, straightforward guide to using natural hormones.

Dr. Lee was a passionate advocate of using commonsense and simple, straightforward solutions to create and maintain optimal health. We felt it was important to write *Hormone Balance Made Simple* because so much of our mail is from women who are aware of their hormonal imbalance and want to get started on a program before delving into the biochemistry of their mood swings and the inner workings of their ovaries. They just want to know, in simple terms, how to use supplemental natural hormones, and how to individualize their hormone regimen for themselves. This book has those answers.

Women also frequently write because they're using natural hormones but don't feel it's helping, or their initial problems eventually return. Asking a few simple questions usually reveals the cause: (1) they're taking too high a dose, (2) their timing is off, or (3) they have constant overwhelming stress in their lives combined with poor eating and exercise habits. This book will also address those issues.

Many women write because they want to use natural hormones with the guidance of their doctor, but the doctor doesn't have the necessary information. I have yet to meet a medical doctor who actually sat down and read *What Your Doctor May Not Tell You About Menopause* who didn't turn on a dime and embrace Dr. Lee's protocol—the concepts are literally that obvious, both intuitively and factually.

This book is in no way a replacement for our other books, *What Your Doctor May Not Tell You About Menopause*, *What Your Doctor May Not Tell You About Premenopause*, and *What Your Doctor May Not Tell You About Breast Cancer*, which are wonderful, intelligent, useful classics that will add greatly to every woman's knowledge and understanding of her body. You will want to refer to the other books for a complete understanding of how and why Dr. Lee's program works if you have a serious hormone-related health problem such as endometriosis, PMS, infertility, breast cancer, or osteoporosis, in order to become educated about the underlying cause. If you're tired all the time and want to know how to support your adrenal glands, then you'll want details on how you can use diet, hormones, and other supplements to get back on your feet. If you suspect that what you're eating is derailing your hormone balance, then you'll want to know in detail how different types of foods can hurt or help. If you've got osteoporosis, then you should be treating it on many levels, from hormones and supplements to specific kinds of exercise. If you've had breast cancer, you'll want to know more about what might have caused it and how to prevent a recurrence. All of this detailed information can be found in our other books, along with hundreds of supporting studies, research, and case histories.

It's notable that since Dr. Lee first wrote his self-published book for doctors back in 1993, hundreds of studies, including the huge and now-famous National Institutes of Health's Women's Health Initiative (WHI), have thoroughly validated his stance on progesterone and conventional hormone replacement therapy. Much of this new research can be found in the revised and updated (2004) edition of *What Your Doctor May* Not *Tell You About Menopause.*

However, if you just want the ABCs of using natural hormones, this is the book for you. Enjoy!

Virginia Hopkins

Introduction

The Life and Work of John R. Lee, M.D.

John R. Lee, M.D., was internationally acknowledged as a pioneer and expert in the study and use of the hormone progesterone, and on the subject of hormone replacement therapy (HRT) for women. He used transdermal (cream rubbed on the skin) progesterone extensively in his clinical practice for nearly a decade, conducting research that showed that it can help reverse osteoporosis.

Dr. Lee died at the age of 73, in October 2003, of a heart attack. He often mused that he felt blessed to have lived so long because many of the men in his family had died of heart attacks in their forties and fifties. His own father, also a medical doctor, died at the age of 49.

Until his death, Dr. Lee kept a full schedule, giving talks and teaching worldwide, and writing his best-selling books and monthly newsletters. Dr. Lee was gratified by the thousands of women who wrote and called to tell him how dramatically their health had improved when they followed his recommendations, and by the hundreds of clinicians and researchers he corresponded with who had integrated his work into their practices and research with great success. Dr. Lee was thankful that his analysis of the problems with conventional HRT were finally validated by the medical establishment during his lifetime. Dr. Lee's wife Pat, and his friends and colleagues will carry on his legacy, as will the millions of others whose lives he touched over the years.

Dr. Lee had a distinguished medical career that included graduating from Harvard and the University of Minnesota Medical School. After he retired from a 30-year family practice in northern California, he began writing and traveling around the world to speak to doctors, scientists, and lay people about progesterone. Dr. Lee also taught a popular course on "Optimal Health" at the College of Marin for 15 years, for which he wrote the book *Optimal Health Guidelines.*

Dr. Lee had a family practice in northern California when, in the early 1970s, he began seeing many menopausal women with health complaints who weren't able to use estrogen because of a high cancer risk, heart disease, or diabetes. About that time he attended a lecture by Raymond Peat, Ph.D., who claimed that estrogen was the wrong hormone to give to menopausal women and that what they really needed was progesterone. Dr. Lee was so influenced by this lecture that he took a list of Dr. Peat's references and checked them out. Sure enough, Dr. Lee became convinced that the research was pointing in a new and important direction in hormone replacement.

Focus on Progesterone

Dr. Lee began recommending that his menopausal patients try using a progesterone cream called Pro-Gest and found they were delighted with the results. These women reported relief from such menopausal symptoms as hot flashes, night sweats, and insomnia, and they also reported relief from a wide array of other symptoms as diverse as dry eyes, bloating, irritability, gallbladder problems, osteoporosis pain, hair loss, and lumpy or sore breasts. As a result of this overwhelmingly positive feedback, Dr. Lee began to collect detailed data on these patients and began to research progesterone more in depth, gathering studies from his local medical library and communicating with scientists around the world to discuss their work. He suspected that progesterone had a positive effect on bone health and ordered bone density tests for his patients who were taking progesterone. Within a few years he realized that these women were gaining significant bone density—particularly the more elderly women who had the lowest bone density to begin with.

What Your Doctor May *Not* Tell You

Dr. Lee was so convinced his clinical experience with progesterone could have a major positive impact on the health of menopausal women that he retired from his family practice and devoted his time to giving talks and writing about natural progesterone. He self-published a book for doctors called *Natural Progesterone: The Multiple Roles of a Remarkable Hormone*, sold it out of his garage, and was soon engaged in a voluminous correspondence with hundreds of women, doctors, and scientists worldwide.

A few years later a medical writer named Virginia Hopkins, who was herself suffering from early menopausal symptoms, came across Dr. Lee's book. She called him to say, "You need to get this information out to the millions of women who are suffering from these symptoms. How about if we do a book together?" Dr. Lee agreed to the plan, and his second book, *What Your Doctor May* Not *Tell You About Menopause*, was published in 1996. This book is a "translation" of the medical language in the first book and expands significantly on the original information. The menopause book sold better than anyone at Warner Books had dreamed it would, and by the fall of 1998 nearly half a million books had sold, almost entirely by word of mouth. The book, now a classic in the genre with over a million copies in print, was extensively rewritten and updated to include research that has come out since the publication of the first edition.

Progesterone Cream Takes Off

Meanwhile, a successful progesterone cream industry was developing, and soon dozens of companies began selling progesterone cream. It literally became a multimillion-dollar industry within a few years. Why? Because progesterone cream really works to alleviate the symptoms of estrogen dominance and menopausal symptoms in general, and conventional medicine has failed to address these concerns in a safe, effective manner. Women have intuitively known for decades that they were being "mistreated" by the medical profession when it came to HRT and have enthusiastically embraced this intuitively obvious and safe solution. Again, the bottom line is that for most women, progesterone supplementation works very well when used as directed, and it is safe. There have been articles claiming that progesterone is not safe, but it is important to note that the research these claims are based on has always been about the synthetic progestins, not on natural progesterone.

Talking to Premenopausal Women from Thirty to Fifty About Hormone Balance

As Dr. Lee traveled around the world giving talks and attending conferences, he soon discovered that at least half of his audience members were premenopausal women from their mid-thirties to late forties. These women suffered from a long list of symptoms, including PMS, fibroids, fibrocystic breasts, weight gain, fatigue, endometriosis, irregular or heavy periods, infertility, and miscarriage, which they intuitively knew were due to hormonal imbalance. When they tried progesterone cream, they often found that it worked wonderfully well to alleviate their symptoms, and Dr. Lee began to collect stacks of mail from women who had avoided hysterectomies, lost weight, had fibroids shrink, found relief from PMS; and some women had finally been able to conceive after years of trying. This experience led him to write the book *What Your Doctor May Not Tell You About Premenopause: Balance Your Hormones and Your Life from Thirty to Fifty.*

The Difficult Subject of Breast Cancer

Another subject that came up repeatedly in Dr. Lee's talks and in his mail was breast cancer. Why was everyone looking at the cure and not the cause? How were hormones involved? Was conventional HRT causing breast cancer? To answer these questions, Dr. Lee and Virginia Hopkins teamed up with breast cancer researcher Dr. David Zava to write *What Your Doctor May Not Tell You About Breast Cancer*. Dr. Zava's many years in the laboratory brought an expertise and depth of knowledge to this book that isn't found elsewhere. Though controversial, this important book challenges the very foundations of the breast cancer industry and carefully explains the underlying causes of breast cancer—from hormonal imbalance and insulin resistance to stress and diet.

Hormone Balance for Men

Along with letters from women about their own health, Dr. Lee received a lot of mail about hormone balance for men. Over the years, he collected research and opinions from clinicians on the subject. Finally in the year before he died, Dr. Lee self-published a booklet called *Hormone Balance for Men*, which is available online at www.johnleemd.com and www.hopkinstestkits.com. This booklet covers such topics as how men's hormones really work, what really causes prostate cancer, and how to safely supplement with natural hormones.

Continuing Dr. Lee's Remarkable Legacy

Dr. Lee's dedication to and research on natural hormone supplementation have changed the lives of millions. Through his books, tapes, videos, and website, he continues to help those seeking hormone balance. His wife, his friends and his colleagues will carry on his remarkable legacy, as will the millions of others whose lives he touched over the years. The most meaningful way to remember John R. Lee, M.D., and carry on his work is to educate others, one-to-one, and give them the gift of optimal health, as he gave us. *Hormone Balance Made Simple* makes Dr. Lee's knowledge more accessible than ever before.

The Hormone Basics

So, you want to try natural hormones. Great! But before you take pills, rub on cream, or apply patches, it's important to know the basics of what you're doing and why. Hormones bring important messages to every cell of your body, with potent results. The hormone imbalances that led you to this book in the first place can be corrected—or made worse—depending on your treatment plan.

For many women, regaining hormone balance is a fairly straightforward matter of using some natural progesterone cream. But for others, whatever created the imbalance in the first place needs to be addressed, and still others have such complicating factors as a hysterectomy, endometriosis, or PMS. This book is designed to help you by giving simple, clear guidelines for creating hormone balance based on your symptoms, lifestyle, and health considerations.

The three basic questions you'll need answered before you can be on your way to hormone balance are:

1. Are my symptoms caused by a hormone imbalance?
2. Which hormones do I need to regain hormone balance?
3. How do I use the hormones for optimal health and balance?

Throughout this book you'll be given the guidelines you need to answer these questions.

Hormones 101

To even talk about hormone balance, there are a few simple concepts that are important to understand. Here's a brief outline of the most important hormones you'll need to know about and how they affect your body. If you'd like more detailed information about any of these hormones, please read our previous books, *What Your Doctor May Not Tell You About Menopause,* or *What Your Doctor May Not Tell You About Premenopause.*

HRT stands for "hormone replacement therapy." In this book, we use the term "conventional HRT" to describe the hormone treatment plans prescribed by doctors for the past 30 years.

Estrogen, progesterone, and testosterone are the three hormones that are most often out of balance in women. They are made by your ovaries and, in much smaller amounts, by your adrenal glands. These three are also called *steroid hormones* or *sex hormones*.

Progesterone helps the female body regulate its menstrual cycles; it's essential for creating and maintaining a pregnancy, it balances the effects of estrogen, and most of your other hormones are made from it.

Estrogen is the hormone that makes you female, endowing you with breasts, hips, menstrual periods, soft skin, and a higher-pitched voice.

Testosterone is the male hormone, but women also make it in small amounts. In women, testosterone primarily contributes to sex drive and helps build bone.

DHEA (dehydroepiandrosterone) is a precursor to testosterone and the estrogens, meaning that those hormones are made from it. DHEA is made primarily in the adrenal glands and is essential for protein building and repair. DHEA levels decline dramatically as we age, making it a primary biomarker of aging.

Androgens are male hormones, including testosterone and androstenedione. DHEA is often considered an androgen but converts readily to estrogen in many women.

Natural or Bioidentical Hormones

Hormones are called *natural* or *bioidentical* if they are exact duplicates of what your body makes. In other words, the molecular structure of a natural hormone is identical to that of the hormones made by your body. This is an important distinction because the hormones typically handed out by your doctor are *not* natural; some of them are completely man-made and are found nowhere in nature, and others, notably Premarin, are made from the urine of pregnant mares. Hormones do very complex and specific jobs in the body by fitting into the part of your cells called receptors, much the same way that a key fits into a lock. Once the hormone is in the receptor, it gives the cell instructions. If the molecular structure is different, *even by one atom*, the instructions given to the cell are different. Hormones that aren't natural to your body give instructions that can be harmful. You'll learn more about which hormones are natural and which aren't later in the book.

Synthetic Hormones

Synthetic hormones are not natural to your body. Drug companies purposely make them different from natural hormones so they can be patented. Patented drugs are important to drug company profits because the company that invents them can sell them exclusively for many years, and thus they can charge more for them because there's no competition. Natural substances cannot be patented and therefore tend to be less expensive. Synthetic hormones are *not* necessarily made, sold, and prescribed because they work better than natural hormones, but because natural hormones can't be patented.

Progestins are synthetic progesterones, used in birth control pills and conventional HRT. Some examples are Provera (medroxyprogesterone acetate), Aygestin (norethindrone acetate), and Megace (megestrol acetate).

Provera is the most commonly used progestin in HRT.

Premarin is an estrogen extracted from pregnant-horse urine. While it is made of natural estrogens, most of them are natural to horses, not humans, which means they have different effects on your body than human estrogens.

PremPro is the most common form of conventional HRT. It is a combination of Premarin and Provera.

Hormone Cycles That Can Lead to Imbalance

Premenopause refers to the years between the ages of 30 and 50 when women's hormones begin to fluctuate and cause such symptoms as PMS, weight gain, endometriosis, fibroids, infertility, and tender breasts, to name a few.

Perimenopause refers to the few years before menopause when many women's hormones are *really* fluctuating, causing even greater weight gain, irregular periods, heavy bleeding, hot flashes, night sweats, insomnia, mood swings, thinning skin, vaginal dryness, loss of sex drive, fatigue, and memory loss.

Menopause is official when you haven't had a menstrual period for one year. Some 95 percent of women reach menopause between the ages of 44 and 55, but the average age of menopause is 50.

Now that you've got the hormone basics, we can move on to Dr. Lee's rules for hormone replacement therapy.

Dr. Lee's Three Rules for Hormone Replacement Therapy

Currently, there are approximately 50 million menopausal women in the United States, and every day about 5,000 more enter menopause. Just a few years ago, most women over the age of 50 who visited their doctors were automatically offered hormone replacement therapy (HRT) whether they seemed to need it or not. As a result, prior to July 2003, an estimated 8 million women were using HRT in the form of PremPro, a cocktail of synthetic hormones. Then the results of a large, government-sponsored study called the Women's Health Initiative (WHI) were released, and they showed that conventional HRT can significantly increase the risk of heart disease, stroke, and breast cancer. It's hard to believe, but the WHI was the first large-scale, long-term study conducted of conventional HRT, which had already been around for decades by the time the study began. The study was halted three years early because after only five years it concluded that conventional HRT could be dangerous.

For 30 years most women had been told by their doctors that they needed HRT after menopause, and now in the wake of this new information about the potential dangers of this treatment, they were being told not to take it. And yet, they were being offered no other solutions for their symptoms, short of antidepressants. Millions of women searched the Internet looking for alternatives, only to find vastly different approaches and opinions, including natural hormones, herbs, vitamins, diets, and the old standby: "Your hormones are fine, you don't need HRT of any kind—just tough it out."

The Natural Hormone Revolution

Meanwhile, over the past decade, hundreds of doctors had begun using natural hormones to help their premenopausal and menopausal patients, and, much to their delight, found that the women they were treating seemed much happier and healthier using the natural hormones than they were using PremPro or other synthetic hormones. A revolution had begun and there was no stopping it. When our first book, *What Your Doctor May* Not *Tell You About Menopause,* was published, it was one of the only books on the subject of using natural hormones, particularly progesterone. Now there are over a million copies of that book in print and there are dozens of books espousing a similar message lining bookstore shelves. That's the good news. The bad news is that there are also a lot of wacky and just plain ignorant ideas out there about how to use natural hormones, some of them, in our opinion, downright dangerous.

The fact is, we don't have any large-scale, double-blind, placebo-controlled, peer-reviewed studies that investigate the safety and efficacy of using natural hormone creams. The closest we have to this type of research is a 10-year observational study conducted in France, that looked at the effects on women of a low-dose estradiol patch plus oral (pill form) progesterone. Women using this combination showed no increased risk of breast cancer, strokes, or heart attacks.

Even though we don't have the large-scale studies, we do have anecdotal evidence, which is to say we have input from hundreds of doctors and their patients. Furthermore, we do know that healthy women naturally produce estrogen, progesterone, and testosterone between puberty and menopause, and it is as safe and effective as Mother Nature can make it. In fact, it is because we know that Mother Nature's approach to natural hormones works that we understand it is important to supplement natural hormones in a way that imitates your own body as closely as reasonably possible. Part of the goal of this book is to show you, in simple steps, exactly how to use natural hormones in a way that is intimately familiar to your body.

Dr. Lee's Three Rules

The following three rules for using supplemental hormones are simple but profound (most profound things are very simple). Dr. Lee's Three Rules form the basis for his entire approach to hormone replacement. Keep these rules in mind and refer back to them as you move toward hormone balance, and you'll always be on the right track. If you have a question about whether you should try something, go back to the rules and see if it works with them.

Later in the book you'll find out how to tell if you're hormone deficient, how to tell the difference between synthetic and bioidentical hormones, and how to arrive at the hormone dose that works best for you.

Dr. Lee's Three Rules for Hormone Replacement Therapy in a Nutshell

Rule 1: Use Hormones Only if You Need Them (e.g., if they are measurably low and/or you have clear symptoms)

Rule 2: Use Bioidentical Hormones Rather Than Synthetic Hormones

Rule 3: Use Hormones Only in Dosages That Create Hormone Balance

Rule 1: Use Hormones Only if You Need Them (e.g., if they are measurably low and/or you have clear symptoms)

You might think this first rule is just plain common sense. After all, we don't give insulin or thyroid hormones to someone unless we have good evidence that they need it. And yet, for years, the majority of conventional physicians routinely prescribed large doses of estrogen and other sex hormones to perimenopausal and menopausal women without finding out whether they were really needed. The assumption was—and still is in many cases—that after menopause, women are automatically hormone deficient. This a false assumption. In fact, some menopausal women may have an excess of some hormones. Much of the rest of this book will be devoted to how to tell if you have a hormone imbalance.

Twenty-five years ago a review of the literature on hormone levels before and after menopause showed that more than two-thirds (66 percent) of women up to age 80 continue to make all the estrogen they need. Since then, the evidence has become stronger. Even with their ovaries removed, women make estrogen in body fat. Women with plenty of body fat may make more estrogen after menopause than slim women make before menopause.

The other common assumption is that using hormones, whether you need them or not, will slow the aging process. Again, not true. All of us are going to continue to age whether or not we're using supplemental hormones. Maintaining hormone *balance* can certainly help slow the process and treat some of the symptoms of aging, but our biological clocks keep on ticking regardless of the pills and potions we take, and that includes hormones.

A majority of women who enter the menopausal transition do not have symptoms bothersome enough to seek medical help. A few irregular periods, a few hot flashes here and there, and it's over. If you're feeling healthy, are at a good weight, eating reasonably well, and getting enough rest and plenty of exercise, chances are that your aging process will be gradual and largely uneventful. If this describes you, then "if it ain't broke, don't fix it" applies.

There's an argument to be made that a little bit of supplemental progesterone can be beneficial to many perimenopausal women and the majority of menopausal women, because we are all awash in a sea of man-made *xenoestrogens*. We are exposed daily to xenoestrogens through plastics and pesticides; through off-gassing from particle board, carpets, and the like; and by our consumption of synthetic hormones in meat and dairy products, just to name a few sources. (See chapter 11 and our other books for details.) This means we carry an unnatural burden of foreign estrogens, and progesterone may help protect us from their effects.

Rule 2: Use Bioidentical (Natural) Hormones Rather Than Synthetic Hormones

Bioidentical hormones are identical to those your body makes. This rule may seem self-evident, but most of the so-called hormones handed out by doctors for the past 30 years are not found in the human body. They should be called pseudo-hormones, or hormone-flavored drugs, because their molecular structure has been altered and they no longer behave exactly like your own hormones. Why would a drug company do such a thing? Because it's more profitable for a drug company to slightly alter the structure of a natural molecule in order to patent it. The patents protect the financial interests of the company, at the expense of women, with natural hormone knock-offs.

How Are Natural Hormone Supplements Made?
Natural hormones are made in a laboratory from soy or wild yams. Even though they're made in a laboratory, they are still the same molecule that your body makes.

How Are Synthetic Hormones Made?
With the notable exception of Premarin, which is a hormone concoction extracted from the urine of pregnant horses, synthetic hormones are also made from soybeans or wild yams (these days most hormones are made from soybeans because they're so inexpensive). In a certain sense the manufacturers of synthetic hormones are taking perfectly good natural hormones and changing their molecular structure to make them unique, not-found-in-nature, so they can be patented. As silly as that idea may seem, it's basically the concept that synthetic hormones are built upon.

Does It Matter Whether Natural Hormones Are Made Out of Soy or Wild Yam?
It makes no difference. By the time the soybeans or wild yams become progesterone, estrogen, or testosterone,

they bear no resemblance to the plant they originate from. It's important to understand that these hormones are not being directly extracted from the plants. There is a substance called diosgenin in soybeans and wild yams that is extracted and then modified in the laboratory to create the hormones. Your body cannot modify diosgenin and turn it into hormones. In other words, you can't take soy or wild yam supplements and expect your hormone levels to change. This can be confusing because soy does contain phytoestrogens, or "plant" estrogens, which can have very mild estrogen-like effects, but these come from a different component of the soybean.

Progesterone and Progestins: What's the Difference?

We have hundreds of letters from women who tell us that their doctor informed them that progesterone and progestins are the same. We suggest that those who still insist that progestins and progesterone are the same, or that progesterone is a generic term that also covers progestins, ponder the following questions. If progesterone and progestins are the same:

▶ Why do fertility doctors always use progesterone and not progestins?

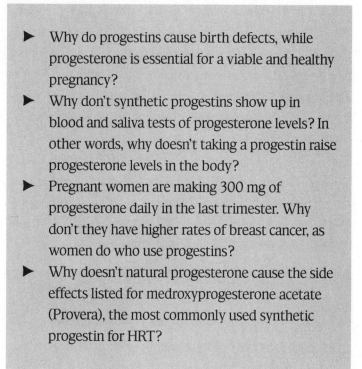

▶ Why do progestins cause birth defects, while progesterone is essential for a viable and healthy pregnancy?

▶ Why don't synthetic progestins show up in blood and saliva tests of progesterone levels? In other words, why doesn't taking a progestin raise progesterone levels in the body?

▶ Pregnant women are making 300 mg of progesterone daily in the last trimester. Why don't they have higher rates of breast cancer, as women do who use progestins?

▶ Why doesn't natural progesterone cause the side effects listed for medroxyprogesterone acetate (Provera), the most commonly used synthetic progestin for HRT?

Suggesting that synthetic, not-found-in-nature hormones will work as well as or better than your own hormones is like saying that breaking down the front door to get inside your home is just as good as putting a key into the lock and turning the knob. You get the same effect of getting inside, but there's a heavy price to pay when you break down the door. The same applies to synthetic hormones. They have *some* of the effects of your own hormones as well as many other negative side effects.

No synthetic hormone provides the same total activity as the natural hormone it is intended to replace, and synthetic hormones often cause undesirable side effects not found with the human hormone. Bioidentical versions—laboratory-synthesized hormones identical to human hormones—have been available for over 50 years.

Rule 3: Use Hormones Only in Dosages That Create Hormone Balance

The third rule is a bit more complicated. Everyone would probably agree that dosages of hormone supplements should restore normal physiologic levels, meaning levels that will create hormone balance.

The question is—how do you define normal physiologic levels? The right dose for one person may not be the right dose for another. Much of this book will guide you through the process of figuring out the right dose for you.

Use Saliva Testing to Get Accurate Hormone Levels

This issue of dosage has been further confused by the conventional blood test, which doesn't provide an accurate picture of available hormones. At any given moment, most of the hormones in your body are unusable—tightly bound to proteins in the bloodstream. Only 1 to 2 percent escape the binding proteins and are free, or bioavailable, to enter tissues throughout the body. Conventional blood tests measure only the total level of hormones in the bloodstream. This is like trying to balance your checkbook without knowing what checks have been paid out.

One of the tissues that bioavailable hormones enter is the saliva gland, and they then freely pass through into the saliva. By collecting saliva and measuring its level of hormones, it is possible to determine the amount of hormones available to other tissues—your current balance. The beauty of saliva testing is that it is available without a prescription and it can be easily collected at home with no poking, pricking, or peeing involved. You just spit into a tube and mail it to the lab.

Hormone replacement therapy is a good approach to optimal health for many women, but it must be done correctly. HRT based on correcting hormone deficiency and restoring proper balance is proposed as a more sane, successful, and safe technique, in contrast to conventional HRT, which violates all three of Dr. Lee's rules.

Other Factors in Hormone Imbalance

Hormone imbalance can be a contributing factor to breast cancer, strokes, and heart attacks. Other risk factors of importance include the following:

Poor diet, including excess sugar and carbohydrates; lack of healthy fats and oils such as the omega-3 fatty acids found in fish; lack of fiber and lack of needed nutrients such as the vitamins and minerals found in healthy foods.

Exposure to toxins such as pesticides and nail polish.

Stress depletes the adrenal glands and by itself can create imbalances among all hormones.

Lifestyle problems such as lack of exercise, excess light at night (causing poor sleep and melatonin deficiency), alcohol, cadmium (cigarette smoking), and using birth control pills during the early teens.

Conventional HRT carries an unacceptable risk of breast cancer, heart attacks, and strokes. A more rational HRT using bioidentical hormones in dosages based on true needs is a more rational approach. Other factors such as lifestyle are all potentially correctable. Combining hormone balancing with correction of other environmental and lifestyle factors is our best hope for reducing the symptoms of hormone imbalance.

The Hormone Balance Test

While a saliva hormone test can give a very accurate picture of which hormones are out of balance, it's always best to compare your results with your symptoms. For that reason, we have devised a Hormone Balance Test that can give you a good sense of which hormones are out of balance, based on your symptoms alone. This was originally created with Dr. David Zava for *What Your Doctor May Not Tell You About Breast Cancer.* It is also available at www.hopkinstestkits.com, where it can be printed out.

Ideally you will be working with a health care professional to both determine which hormones are out of balance and to create a protocol using natural hormones to bring your body back into balance.

1. Read carefully through the list of symptoms in each group, and put a check mark next to each

symptom that you have. (If you check off the same symptom in more than one group, that's fine.)

2. Go back and count the check marks in each group. In any group where you have two or more symptoms checked off, there's a good chance that you have the hormone imbalance represented by that group.

3. The more symptoms you check off, the higher the likelihood that you have the hormone imbalance represented by that group. (Some people may have more than one type of hormonal imbalance.)

Symptom Group 1

☐ PMS
☐ Insomnia
☐ Early miscarriage
☐ Painful and/or lumpy breasts
☐ Unexplained weight gain
☐ Cyclical headaches
☐ Anxiety
☐ Infertility
____ TOTAL BOXES CHECKED

Symptom Group 2

☐ Vaginal dryness
☐ Night sweats
☐ Painful intercourse
☐ Memory problems
☐ Bladder infections
☐ Lethargic depression
☐ Hot flashes
____ TOTAL BOXES CHECKED

Symptom Group 3

☐ Puffiness and bloating
☐ Cervical dysplasia (abnormal pap smear)
☐ Rapid weight gain
☐ Breast tenderness
☐ Mood swings
☐ Heavy bleeding
☐ Anxious depression
☐ Migraine headaches
☐ Insomnia
☐ Foggy thinking
☐ Red flush on face
☐ Gallbladder problems
☐ Weepiness
____ TOTAL BOXES CHECKED

30

Symptom Group 4

A combination of the symptoms in group 1 and group 3. (If you have checked two or more boxes in each of these two groups, you may belong to symptom group 4.)

____ TOTAL BOXES CHECKED

Symptom Group 5

- ☐ Acne
- ☐ Polycystic ovary syndrome (PCOS)
- ☐ Excessive hair on the face and the arms
- ☐ Hypoglycemia and/or unstable blood sugar
- ☐ Thinning hair on the head
- ☐ Infertility
- ☐ Ovarian cysts
- ☐ Mid-cycle pain

____ TOTAL BOXES CHECKED

Symptom Group 6

- ☐ Debilitating fatigue
- ☐ Unstable blood sugar
- ☐ Foggy thinking
- ☐ Low blood pressure
- ☐ Thin and/or dry skin
- ☐ Intolerance to exercise
- ☐ Brown spots on face

____ TOTAL BOXES CHECKED

If you have checked two or more boxes in one or more symptom groups, see the "Answers" section below to find out what type of hormonal imbalance(s) you may have.

Answers

Symptom Group 1
Progesterone deficiency: This is the most common hormone imbalance among women of all ages. You may need to change your diet, eliminate synthetic hormones (including birth control pills), and begin to use some progesterone cream.

Symptom Group 2
Estrogen deficiency: This hormone imbalance is most common in menopausal women—especially if you are petite and/or slim. You may need to make some special changes to your diet or take some women's herbs (see our ... *Premenopause* book); some women may even need a little bit of natural estrogen (about one-tenth the dose usually prescribed by doctors).

Symptom Group 3
Excess estrogen: In women, this is most often solved by getting off of the conventional synthetic hormones most often prescribed by doctors for menopausal

women. Adding progesterone often helps relieve symptoms and balance hormones.

Symptom Group 4

Estrogen dominance: This is caused when you don't have enough progesterone to balance the effects of estrogen. Thus, you can have low estrogen or symptoms of estrogen deficiency, but if you have even lower progesterone, you can have symptoms of estrogen dominance. Many women between the ages of 40 and 50 suffer from estrogen dominance. You may want to try using some natural progesterone cream. In saliva hormone testing, when your estrogen is at its optimal level, your progesterone should be about 200 times higher. In other words, the ratio of progesterone to estrogen for hormone balance would be about 200:1.

Symptom Group 5

Excess androgens (male hormones): This is most often caused by too much sugar and simple carbohydrates in the diet, and can often be changed with simple dietary changes and regular, moderate exercise. Detailed diet and exercise information can be found in our previous books.

Symptom Group 6

Cortisol deficiency: This is caused by tired adrenals, which is usually caused by chronic stress. If you're trying to juggle a job and a family, chances are good you have tired adrenals. Please read either *What Your Doctor May Not Tell You About Menopause* or *What Your Doctor May Not Tell You About Premenopause* for detailed recommendations on restoring tired adrenals.

A Word About Thyroid Deficiency and Hormone Balance

Thyroid hormone levels are closely tied to sex hormone balance. For example, excess estrogen can block thyroid function. If your hormone imbalance symptoms have largely resolved and your saliva test shows normal hormone levels, yet you have cold hands and feet, a lack of stamina, brittle nails and dry hair, you may be suffering from a thyroid deficiency. If you suspect this may be the case, we recommend that you find a doctor who specializes in thyroid function and have your thyroid hormone levels tested.

Now that you have a better idea of which of your hormones may be out of balance, you can read up on how to go about correcting those imbalances. In the next chapter you'll receive guidelines for tracking your symptoms, and later in the book you'll read about timing and dosage information that can help you zero in on what's right for you as an individual. We hope that you'll use the information from this book and our other books to work with your health care professional to create a hormone balance program that's optimal for your body.

Tracking and Interpreting Your Symptoms

Your most powerful ally in your goal of hormone balance and optimal health is yourself! Although it is ideal if you can work with a qualified health care professional, ultimately it's up to you to educate yourself and keep track of how you're doing. It can be very helpful to observe your symptoms before you start using natural hormones and for at least a few months after you begin. If you find that some of your symptoms are returning, you can start tracking them again.

Maintaining hormone balance is more than just taking the right hormones in the correct timing and dosage. Many aspects of your lifestyle, from diet and exercise to stress and sleep patterns, can impact hormone levels.

Good health and hormone balance are a reflection of how you are doing on each level of human consciousness: physical, emotional, mental, and spiritual. To truly assess where to make the changes that lead to optimal health and well-being, it's wise to address each level. Emotional, mental, and spiritual turmoil are frequently at the root of the hormone imbalances that lead to physical problems. For example, at the spiritual level, a sense of disconnectedness from God (or whatever your higher power or purpose is) can lead to mental and emotional turmoil that manifests as depression, worry, fear, obsessiveness, overwork, and conflict in relationships. These states of consciousness often spill over into poor lifestyle choices such as eating junk food, lack of exercise, and drug and alcohol abuse, which in turn cause the chronic health problems we're all too familiar with, such as diabetes, heart disease, arthritis—and hormone imbalances. Going within and addressing the sense of disconnectedness can begin a positive transformation that leads to addressing the mental and emotional turmoil, which in turn leads to better lifestyle choices, which leads to hormone balance. Using supplemental hormones without addressing the other levels of consciousness may only solve the problem temporarily, or health problems may pop up in other areas of the body.

The symptom checklist on pages 38–39 will help you

Keep Track of Your Symptoms: Symptom Checklist

Symptom　　　　Days	1	2	3	4	5	6	7	8	9	10	11	12	13
Aches and pains													
Acne, oily skin													
Allergies													
Anxiety													
Breast tenderness													
Cold hands and feet													
Decreased sex drive													
Depression													
Dry eyes													
Dry skin													
Dry, brittle hair													
Endometriosis													
Fat gain													
Fatigue													
Fibrocystic (lumpy) breasts													
Foggy thinking													
Gallbladder pain													
Hair loss													
Headaches													
Heart palpitations													
Hot flashes													
Hypoglycemia (low blood sugar)													
Incontinence													
Insomnia (inability to sleep)													
Irritability													
Memory loss													
Migraines													
Muscle weakness													
Night sweats													
Osteoporosis													
Ovarian cysts													
Oversensitivity													
Painful intercourse													
PMS													
Sleepiness													
Sluggish digestion													
Talking excessively													
Thinning skin													
Urinary tract irritation and/or infection													
Uterine fibroids													
Vaginal dryness													
Water retention, bloating													
Weepiness													
Weight gain													

14	15	16	17	18	19	20	21	22	23	24	25	26	27	28	29	30

play detective for yourself and find out which symptoms are the most frequent and troublesome.

You can print out a copy of this list at www .hopkinstestkits.com and use it to create a chart for yourself that tracks the symptoms you have. Rate your symptoms on a scale of 0 to 5 so that you can easily see over time how you're doing.

0: Not a problem
1: Rarely a problem
2: Bothers me occasionally
3: Regularly a problem
4: Almost always a problem
5: Constantly a problem

Ideally you should track your symptoms every day for a month if you're premenopausal, and for two weeks if you're menopausal, before starting on hormone supplements, and then continue for at least three months. If you find that some of your symptoms aren't improving, check the list of possible causes that begins on page 43.

Keep a Lifestyle Journal

Many factors can derail your hormone balance. It can be very helpful to keep a lifestyle journal for a month, to find out if something unexpected in your life is adversely affecting your health (or for that matter, if something unexpected is improving your health!). Here are some of the lifestyle factors to track:

Breakfast
Lunch
Dinner
Snacks
Beverages
Glasses of water
Vitamins/supplements
Bedtime (what time did you go to bed?)
Hours of sleep
Exercise
Recreation (movies, parties, etc.)
Stress level (on a scale of 1 to 5 with 5 the highest)
What was the stressor?
Prescription drugs
Over-the-counter drugs
Exposure to toxins (e.g., smog, car exhaust, glue, acetone, nail polish, bug spray, new house, new furniture or carpet, perfume, air "fresheners")
TV watching
TV news watching
Relationships with others (on a scale of 1 to 5 with 5 being ideal)

Specific Symptoms and Related Hormone Imbalances

Many health care professionals who work with natural hormones use symptoms exclusively (versus testing blood, urine, and saliva levels) to arrive at a treatment plan. While the Hormone Balance Test in chapter 3 gives you a good general overview of which hormonal imbalance may be causing your symptoms, the following list of symptoms and their possible causes is much more detailed, to help you narrow in on underlying causes.

Two Reminders: (1) Estrogen dominance means there's not enough progesterone to balance the effects of estrogen. Thus, you may have estrogen deficiency symptoms and your estrogen may measure low, but if you have low progesterone you can still have estrogen dominance symptoms. Your estrogen may also be normal, but if you don't have progesterone to balance it, you can have estrogen dominance symptoms. (2) If you used natural hormones for a few months and found that your symptoms returned, it's usually because: (a) you're taking too high a dose, (b) your timing is off, or (c) you have constant overwhelming stress in your life combined with poor eating, sleeping, and exercise habits.

Symptoms and Their Possible Causes

- **Aches and Pains**

  Low cortisol
  Estrogen dominance
  Low testosterone

- **Acne, Oily Skin**

  High testosterone (see ovarian cysts)

- **Allergies**

  Estrogen dominance
  Low cortisol
  Deficiency of vitamin C and bioflavonoids (eat
    more fresh fruits and veggies)

- **Anxiety**

  Estrogen dominance
  Too much caffeine (coffee, soft drinks, etc.)
  Diet pills
  Deficiency of B vitamins
  Chronic stress
  Too much TV

- **Breast Tenderness**

  Estrogen dominance
  Too much caffeine
  Supplementing with estrogen, testosterone,

DHEA, or pregnenolone can create excess
estrogen and cause breast tenderness.

- **Cold Hands and Feet**

  Estrogen dominance interfering with thyroid
  function
  Low thyroid
  Poor circulation caused by excess sugar in the diet
  Insulin resistance

- **Decreased Sex Drive**

  Low testosterone
  Estrogen dominance
  Stress

- **Depression**

  Both high and low estrogen can contribute to
  depression.
  Low progesterone

- **Dry Eyes**

  Estrogen dominance
  Low testosterone

- **Dry Skin**

  Estrogen deficiency
  Estrogen dominance creating low thyroid function

- **Dry, Brittle Hair**

  Estrogen dominance creating low thyroid function
  Low progesterone

- **Endometriosis**

  Probably caused by exposure to xenoestrogens
  (estrogens that are foreign to the body, such
  as are found in pesticides and plastics) in the
  womb and made worse by estrogen dominance

Abdominal Fat

In menopausal women, estrogen is both made and
maintained by belly fat. This would explain why, in
middle age, even slim women get a bit of a belly—
nature's way of making sure we get what we need.
However, a too-fat abdomen is not good for the
heart. At what point (or at what size) does "good"
belly fat become "bad" belly fat? It's quite natural for
a postmenopausal woman to have a little bit of a
belly, but more than that is usually an indicator of
insulin resistance and/or high cortisol. The best way
to tell whether it's helpful or harmful is simply by
how it looks—an insulin-resistant belly is noticeably
out of proportion to the rest of the body even in
someone who is obese.

- **Fat Gain**

  Excess fat around the hips, buttocks, and thighs is a hallmark symptom of estrogen dominance.

  Excess fat around the middle is usually a sign of insulin resistance (too much sugar and refined carbohydrates, too little exercise).

  A poochy tummy (which is different from weight gain around the middle, and different from the saggy tummy caused by pregnancy) can be caused by excess cortisol (stress), and/or estrogen deficiency, and/or constipation.

- **Fatigue**

  Low cortisol

  Estrogen dominance

  Stress

  Lack of sleep

  Chronic infection

  Poor diet (which can cause hypoglycemia, a condition where blood sugar drops dramatically between meals)

- **Fibrocystic (lumpy) Breasts**

  Estrogen dominance (Progesterone cream applied directly to the breasts almost always clears this up.)

Supplementing with estrogen, testosterone, DHEA, or pregnenolone can create excess estrogen and cause lumpy breasts.

- **Foggy Thinking**

  Low estrogen
  Low testosterone
  Estrogen dominance
  Hypoglycemia (low blood sugar)

- **Gallbladder Pain**

  Excess estrogen
  Estrogen dominance
  Too much fat in the diet (especially fried foods)

- **Hair Loss**

  Excess testosterone/male hormones (usually caused by excess sugar and refined carbohydrates in the diet)
  Excess estrogen
  Estrogen dominance
  Thyroid deficiency

- **Headaches**

  Estrogen dominance

- **Heart Palpitations**

  Low cortisol

  Low testosterone

  Low blood pressure

  Food allergy

  Stress

- **Hot Flashes**

  Low estrogen

  Low progesterone

  Fluctuating hormones caused by the menopausal transition

- **Hypoglycemia (low blood sugar)**

  Estrogen dominance

  Low cortisol

- **Incontinence (e.g., I wet my pants when I laugh, cough, or sneeze)**

  Overall low hormones; especially common among women with hysterectomy

  Obesity

- **Insomnia (can't get to sleep and/or wake up a lot)** It is not at all unusual for women going through the menopausal transition to experience some sleep disturbances, with or without supplemental hormones. For most it passes within a year. Progesterone is a calming hormone, and applying some at night before bed can help quite a bit.

Estrogen dominance

Excess estrogen

Too much caffeine

Too much light in the room

Excess cortisol (e.g., stress, worries)

- **Irritability**

  Low estrogen

  Estrogen dominance

  High testosterone ("testiness")

  Excess cortisol (e.g., stress)

- **Memory loss**

  Stress (high cortisol can cause short-term memory loss)

  Low estrogen

  Estrogen dominance

- **Migraines (especially premenstrual)**

  Estrogen dominance

- **Muscle Weakness**

  Low cortisol

  Low testosterone

  Low progesterone

- **Night Sweats**

  Low estrogen

  Estrogen dominance

  Low progesterone

  Fluctuating estrogens caused by the menopausal transition

- **Osteoporosis**

  Low progesterone (progesterone helps build bone)

  Low testosterone (testosterone helps build bone)

  Low estrogen (estrogen helps slow bone loss)

  Excess cortisol

- **Ovarian Cysts**

  Often caused by too much sugar and refined carbs in the diet, which raises insulin levels, which stimulates the ovaries to produce more androgens (male hormones), which cause ovarian cysts. One of the simplest (if not easiest) hormone imbalances to fix with good food and plenty of exercise.

- **Oversensitivity**

  Excess estrogen

- **Painful Intercourse**

  Low estrogen

  Low testosterone

Insulin and PCOS

Many young women have polycystic ovary syndrome (PCOS), where cysts on the ovaries cause pain during ovulation, PMS, and excess hair growth on the face, legs, and arms. It's been known for some time that PCOS is associated with high insulin levels, which stimulate the ovarian production of androgens (male hormones). In a study of obese and non-obese women with PCOS (Nobumasa et al., *Reproductive Medicine and Technology* 2002), various hormones were measured with interesting results.

Researchers measured blood levels of six markers, including estradiol, testosterone, and androstenedione. The average levels of testosterone and androstenedione in obese PCOS women were significantly higher than those in non-obese PCOS women.

This is yet another indicator that obesity can contribute significantly to hormone imbalance. PCOS disappears rapidly in most women when they cut sugar and refined carbohydrates from their diet.

- **PMS**

  Estrogen dominance

- **Sleepiness**

  Excess progesterone (applies only to a gross overdose, most often seen with oral progesterone)

  Lack of sleep (this may seem obvious, but the majority of Americans don't get enough sleep)

- **Sluggish Digestion**

  Excess progesterone (applies only to gross overdose, most often seen with oral progesterone)

  Thyroid deficiency

- **Talking Excessively**

  Excess estrogen

  Excess cortisol (stress)

- **Thinning Skin**

  Very high or very low cortisol

  Low testosterone

  Low estrogen

- **Urinary Tract Irritation and/or Infection**

  Low estrogen

  Bacterial infection

  Loss of "good" bacteria caused by antibiotic use

- **Uterine Fibroids**

  Unknown cause, but made worse by estrogen dominance. When they get larger, exposure to excess estrogen or progesterone can cause them to grow.

- **Vaginal Dryness**

  Low estrogen
  Low testosterone

- **Water Retention, Bloating, Puffiness**

  Estrogen dominance
  Excess estrogen

- **Weepiness**

  Estrogen dominance
  Stress
  Depression

- **Weight Gain**

  Estrogen dominance
  Too much sugar and refined carbohydrates in the diet
  Lack of exercise
  Low thyroid

This chapter can be useful for both tracking your symptoms and identifying some of the causes of your symptoms. It's much easier to correct a health problem when you're aware of the underlying cause. Although many women—particularly in partnership with a health care professional—can identify the source of their hormone imbalance by tracking symptoms and identifying their underlying causes, others prefer to get some hard data by actually testing hormone levels. The next chapter will introduce you to some of the ins and outs of testing your hormone levels.

Testing Your Hormone Levels

The most common way to test hormone levels has been with a blood test that measures the hormone levels in the watery blood serum or blood plasma. This is called the serum level. In our opinion, these tests are not very useful because they don't measure your bioavailable "free" hormones accurately. Blood tests can be particularly misleading when measuring hormone levels in a woman who is using transdermal (cream, gel) progesterone. Dr. David Zava explains:

> When the ovaries produce progesterone and it enters the bloodstream, about 98 percent of it is tightly bound to proteins in the bloodstream, and is not

"free" to move into the tissues of the body. In contrast, when hormones are delivered through the skin and enter the bloodstream, a much higher percentage are bioavailable. This shows up in tissues such as those in the salivary gland and then in saliva. Hormones delivered through the skin don't accumulate in the bloodstream because they are efficiently delivered to tissues. This is why a daily dose of 15 to 30 mg [milligrams] of progesterone cream results in a very small increase (if at all) on a blood test, but a significant increase in a saliva test. The information you need to determine your hormone balance is how much hormone is entering your tissues.

Saliva Testing

Saliva testing is quicker, less expensive, and less painful than blood tests, and is a reliable way for your doctor to measure hormone levels and test for hormone deficiencies. This test will confirm that the hormones you are taking are being absorbed and utilized; it doesn't involve a trip to a lab or drawing blood; and it's inexpensive enough that you can do a number of tests—for instance, several over the course of a day or a month. For those women who wish to monitor their own hormone levels to find out if they are ovulating, for example, the tests can be ordered and easily done at home without a doctor's prescription.

When you get the results of a saliva test, the normal range of estradiol in a premenopausal woman is 1.5 to 3 picograms per milliliter (pg/ml), and in a menopausal woman is usually about half that, 1 to 1.5 pg/ml of estradiol. The healthy ratio of progesterone to estradiol is at least 200 to 1 and can go up to 1,000 to 1 in women using transdermal (delivered through the skin with cream, gels, oils) progesterone. Therefore, you would want the saliva progesterone level to be at least 200 pg/ml in a menopausal woman with an estradiol level of about 1 to 1.5 and even higher in a premenopausal woman with an estradiol level of 1.5 to 3 pg/ml.

When estradiol is lower than the optimal range and symptoms indicate an ongoing estrogen deficiency, it is often helpful to try estrogen replacement. Because estrogen and progesterone functions are interrelated, correcting an estrogen deficiency can also help you get optimal benefit from supplemental progesterone.

Normal or optimal ranges of hormones in saliva vary according to whether you're premenopausal, perimenopausal, menopausal, or using some form of HRT. When you take the test, which involves spitting into one or more tubes and mailing them to the lab, your results will be compared to optimal ranges for your age and menopausal status.

Blood Serum or Plasma Testing

When your doctor orders a standard blood test to measure your hormone levels, it's a test of the serum (the watery part of the blood). Serum levels of progesterone will rise to about 2 to 4 nanograms per milliliter (ng/ml) in most women using 20 to 30 mg of progesterone cream. If your doctor measures your serum progesterone levels, here are some guidelines:

- Normal, untreated (not on HRT) menopausal women will show an initial serum progesterone level that is less than 0.5 ng/ml.
- After using progesterone cream, progesterone levels usually rise to 2 to 4 ng/ml.
- In normal *pre*menopausal women, luteal (mid-cycle) phase serum progesterone levels are 4 to 20 ng/ml.

Saliva testing is an inexpensive, uninvasive, and easy way to get an accurate reading of your hormone levels in order to determine whether your estradiol, or progesterone, or testosterone level is in a healthy range. If you get a saliva test of these three hormones once or twice a year, you'll have a good indicator of whether your hormones are in balance.

Getting Off Conventional HRT and On Natural Hormones

The Women's Health Initiative (WHI), the largest government study of synthetic hormones, was halted prematurely in July 2003 (it was originally planned to continue for three more years) because early results indicated that women using conventional HRT (specifically PremPro) had a significantly increased risk of invasive breast cancer, heart disease, and stroke. The study analyzed the health of 16,000 women aged 50 to 79 years old. After five years, those using HRT (Premarin and Provera or PremPro) were estimated to have a 29 percent higher risk of breast cancer, a 26 percent higher risk of heart disease, and a 41 percent higher risk of stroke.

To personalize these numbers a bit more, let's project them out into the general population: Of the 6 million women who were reportedly estimated to be using Prem-Pro at the time, this would translate to approximately 4,200 women who would get breast cancer, 4,800 women who would get heart disease, and 10,800 women who would have a stroke in a five-year period because they were taking this form of HRT. If we extend these numbers out over a decade, nearly 40,000 women would be harmed (many of them killed) by taking these drugs. That's an epidemic, and it doesn't include all the women who suffered from many of the debilitating side effects of using synthetic hormones such as weight gain, fatigue, depression, irritability, headaches, insomnia, bloating, low thyroid, low libido, gallbladder disease, and blood clots.

The results of the WHI study data on breast cancer were confirmed in August 2003 by the publication in the prestigious medical journal *The Lancet* of the first results of the "Million Women Study," which involved around 1 million women over the age of 50 in the United Kingdom. The authors of this study concluded that: "Use of HRT by women aged 50–64 years in the UK over the past decade has resulted in an estimated 20,000 extra breast cancers, 15,000 associated with oestrogen-progestagen [estrogen-progestin]; the extra deaths cannot be reliably estimated."

It's a Matter of Using the *Right* HRT

A relatively large 10-year study from France (*Climacteric* 2002;5:332–340) provides excellent clinical evidence that using natural progesterone does not increase breast cancer risk. In it, B. de Lignieres and colleagues compared different categories of HRT but this time included progesterone (oral or pill form as it happened). They found that women who were on long-term HRT using topical estradiol gel (in much smaller doses than when taken orally) and oral progesterone had no increased risk of breast cancer compared to non-users.

They concluded that there is no reason not to use HRT made of estradiol gel and progesterone, and they regard this type of HRT to be "beneficial for quality of life, prevention of bone loss and cardiovascular risk profile, without the activation of coagulation and inflammatory protein synthesis measured in users of oral estrogen." This is a good step, we believe, in showing that progesterone is much better than Provera when used in HRT, and that lower dose topical (creams, gels, patches) estradiol is better than oral estradiol.

Small studies published since then of women using progesterone cream with or without estrogen are showing positive results. For example, a study by Kenna Stephenson, M.D., and others, at the College of Nursing and

Health Sciences at the University of Texas at Tyler, showed evidence that natural progesterone cream provides relief for the symptoms of menopause while showing no short-term health risks. The study examined the short-term effect of topical progesterone cream on menopausal symptom relief in 30 healthy postmenopausal women and was published in the journal *Blood* in the November 16, 2004, issue. The authors concluded that "admin-istration of topical progesterone cream at a daily dose of 20 mg significantly relieves menopausal symptoms in postmenopausal women without adversely altering pro-thrombotic potential [e.g., increasing the risk of stroke]. Since the thrombotic complications that are typically ob-served with conventional hormone replacement therapy do not seem to occur with topical progesterone, this treat-ment should be seriously considered as an effective and safe alternative clinical therapy for women suffering from menopausal symptoms."

The real point made by these studies is that the safety and efficacy of HRT depends on what kind of HRT is being used. It's not a matter of HRT or no HRT, it's a mat-ter of using the right HRT.

Questions and Answers About Switching to Bioidentical Hormones

Q: Do the results of the WHI apply to your recommendations of using natural estrogen and progesterone?

A: Not at all. What I recommend is first measuring saliva hormone levels and/or tracking symptoms to find if there is a hormonal imbalance. Then, if necessary, correct the imbalance using natural hormones in physiologic doses, which means ordinary doses that the body would naturally produce itself. Another way to look at this is, from puberty until menopause, a healthy woman's body is making its own natural hormones in synchrony and balance, without giving her cancer, heart disease, or strokes. What I recommend is attempting to regain this natural balance as closely as possible. I also believe that because we are exposed on a daily basis to so many man-made xenoestrogens, progesterone may help offset their effects (see chapter 11 and our other books for details).

Conventional HRT not only fails to measure hormones and use physiologic doses, it uses synthetic, not-found-in-nature "hormones" that are foreign to the human body and cause a long list of unwanted side effects.

Q: How do I get off of PremPro and other synthetic HRT drugs?

A. Most women simply need to lower their dose of estrogen and replace the progestin (the "pro" part of the Prem-Pro) with progesterone cream.

Estrogen is a prescription-only medication in the United States, so you'll need to ask your doctor for a separate prescription for estrogen, preferably either estradiol, or a combination of estradiol and estriol, or estriol alone (see table on pages 68–69). If you discontinue estrogen suddenly, you're likely to suffer from hot flashes and night sweats. Hot flashes and night sweats are less likely if the estrogen dose is decreased very gradually.

Unless your doctor already has you on a low dose of estrogen, you can begin with half the dose you have been taking when you add progesterone cream in place of the progestin.

PremPro Doses

High dose: 0.625 mg of Premarin and 2.5 mg of
    Provera (and above)

Medium dose: 0.45 mg of Premarin and 1.5 mg
    of Provera

Low dose: 0.3 mg of Premarin and 1.5 mg of
    Provera

Remember, Premarin is the estrogen part of the formula. In the past, the majority of women were offered the 0.625 dose, but in response to the WHI study, most women who are still using Premarin are now offered one of the lower doses.

Many menopausal women don't need any estrogen at all and can gradually taper (over three to four months) their dose down to nothing. The more fat you have on your body, the more estrogen you're making and the less likely it is that you will need to supplement with estrogen.

Although transdermal progesterone alone will alleviate menopausal symptoms for many women, some may need a little bit of estrogen to control their symptoms. The most common symptoms of estrogen deficiency include hot flashes, night sweats, vaginal dryness, and sleep disturbances. (See chapter 4 for details.)

Natural/Bioidentical HRT vs. Synthetic HRT

Many doctors are confused about what's a natural hormone and what's a synthetic hormone. The only HRT hormones that are natural to humans are estradiol, estrone, estriol, progesterone, and testosterone. Progesterone is available over the counter (e.g., without a prescription). Androstenedione and DHEA are natural hormones that are available over the counter, but since they are often converted into estrogen in the body, it's not advisable to use them without the guidance of a health care professional and/or regular saliva hormone level tests.

(Natural/Bioidentical HRT vs. Synthetic HRT, continued)

For clarification, the available forms (pills, creams, patches, etc.) and dosage strengths of synthetic HRT drugs and natural/ bioidentical HRT are listed below.

SYNTHETIC HRT DRUGS

Oral (Pill Form) Estrogens

Premarin

0.3 mg, 0.625 mg, 0.9 mg, 1.25 mg, 2.5 mg, 0.45 mg

Ogen (estropipate)

0.625 mg, 1.25 mg, 2.5 mg

Ortho-Est (estropipate)

0.625 mg, 1.25 mg

Menest (esterfied)

0.3 mg, 0.625 mg, 1.25 mg, 2.5 mg

Cenestin (synthetic conjugated estrogen)

0.625 mg, 0.9 mg, 1.25 mg

Estinyl (synthetic estrogen)

0.02 mg, 0.05 mg, 0.5 mg

Estrogen/Progestin Combinations (Pills and Patches)

$$\left(\begin{array}{l} \text{NA = norethindrone acetate, a progestin} \\ \text{CEE = conjugated equine estrogens, e.g., Premarin} \\ \text{MPA = medroxyprogesterone acetate} \end{array} \right)$$

Activella   1 mg 17B-estradiol
                    + 0.5 mg norethindrone acetate (NA)

Combipatch	0.05 mg 17B-estradiol + 0.25 mg or 0.05 mg 17B-estradiol + 0.14 mg NA
Climarapro	0.045 mg 17 estradiol with 0.015 mg of levonorgestrel
Femhrt	5 mcg ethinyl estadiol + 1 mg NA
Prefest	1 mg 17B-estradiol for 3 days, alternating with 1 mg 17B-estradiol + 0.09 mg NA for 3 days
PremPro	0.625 mg CEE + 5 mg MPA or 0.625 mg CEE + 2.5 mg MPA
PremPro Low Dose	0.45 mg CEE + 1.5 mg MPA or 0.3 mg CEE + 1.5 mg MPA
Premphase	0.625 mg CEE (alone days 1–14) followed by 0.625 mg CEE + 5.0 mg MPA (days 15–28)

Forms of Oral (Pill Form) Mexdroxyprogesterone Acetate (MPA) (e.g., Provera)

Provera	5 mg, 10 mg, 2.5 mg, 1.5 mg days 1–12
Amen	10 mg days 1–12
MPA	1.5 mg (for use with lower doses of Premarin)

Estrogen/Testosterone Combinations (Pills and Patches)

Estratest	1.25 mg esterfied estrogens, 2.5 mg methyltestosteronegen

(Natural/Bioidentical HRT vs. Synthetic HRT, continued)

Premarin with Methyltestosterone	0.625 Premarin, and 1.25 mg, 5 mg, 10 mg methyltestosterone

NATURAL/BIOIDENTICAL HRT HORMONES

Estrogen Creams

Estrace Cream (estradiol)	0.1 mg estradiol per 1 gram of cream, 1 to 2 grams daily
* **Bi-Est** (estradiol, estriol)	one part estradiol to four parts estriol
* **Tri-Est** (estrone, estradiol, estriol)	one part estrone (E1), to one part estradiol (E2), to 8 parts estriol (E3)

Estrogen Patches

Alora, Climara, Esclim, Estraderm, Vivelle, Vivelle-Dot
(estradiol) 0.025 to 0.1 mg

Oral (Pill Form) Estrogens

Estrace (estradiol) 0.5 mg, 1 mg, 2 mg

Vaginal Estrogens

Estring (Intravaginal Ring) 7.5 mcg (micrograms) daily
(estradiol)

Femring (Intravaginal Ring) (estradiol)	50 mcg or 100 mcg daily
Vagifem Tablets (estradiol)	25 mcg daily for 2 weeks, then 25 mcg 2 times per week
Estrace vaginal cream (estradiol)	0.1 mg estradiol per gram of cream
Progesterone	
Prometrium (oral/pill)	100 mg, 200 mg
Crinone (vaginal cream)	4%, 8% progesterone gel
Progesterone Cream	Dozens available over-the-counter, on the Internet, and from compounding pharmacists

* Made to individual specifications by compounding pharmacists

Q: My doctor says that I can't use estrogen and progesterone cream, because progesterone cream won't protect my uterus the way the progestins do.

A: Progesterone cream does protect the uterus. No problems were found or reported by the hundreds of menopausal patients in my practice before I retired. After my retirement, I remained in touch with dozens of physicians who have thousands of patients among them who have also not reported problems (some of them have been doing this for more than a decade). Furthermore, two double-blind, placebo-controlled studies by Helen Leonetti, M.D., prove that progesterone cream protects the uterus. Her study compared the uterine protection of PremPro (Premarin and Provera) with the same dose of Premarin combined with topical progesterone instead of Provera. In short, the women on the progesterone cream were well protected against estrogen-induced endometrial cancer.

You might also ask your doctor how your *premeno-pausal* body protected itself against estrogen effects! It was not a progestin, it was the *natural* progesterone made by your ovaries every month.

Q: My doctor says that because blood tests don't show a rise in progesterone when progesterone cream is used, it doesn't work, and I should use oral progesterone.

A: Blood tests measure only the serum, which is the watery part of the blood, and progesterone that enters the body from a transdermal cream goes almost directly into your tissues and saliva. Since it does not accumulate in the bloodstream or serum, the most accurate way to measure the hormone in your tissues is with a saliva hormone level test (see chapter 5 for details).

Q: I read an article in a major magazine where a doctor is quoted as saying that natural progesterone stimulates tissue growth in the breast and therefore could contribute to breast cancer. Is this true?

A: We have tracked down the source of this information, and once again, it was a progestin, not progesterone, that stimulated the cell growth in the study being referred to. As you'll read in our books, progesterone first stimulates cells to grow toward differentiation, which is an *anti*-cancer property, and then inhibits further estrogen-stimulated cell growth. Cancer cells are undifferentiated and thus grow without control. Progesterone also encourages cells to die when they're supposed to (which cancer cells don't do). This topic is covered in detail in *What Your Doctor May Not Tell You About Breast Cancer.*

Q: I am soon to turn 51 and have been on Premarin 0.625 mg and medroxyprogesterone [Provera] 2.5 mg for the past two years. I take one tablet of Premarin daily and one tablet of medroxyprogesterone the last 12 days of the month. I just ordered some progesterone cream and a phytoestrogen made from red clover extract. How do I wean myself off the Premarin and medroxyprogesterone and get on these natural products the correct way?

A: I recommend that you stop the medroxyprogesterone immediately and start the progesterone cream. However, that is likely a dose of Premarin that is higher than needed for most women, and your brain becomes, in effect, addicted to the high levels of estrogen. This is because estrogen stimulates the brain, and excess estrogen overstimulates the brain. Estrogen also appears to be tied into the production of serotonin and dopamine, both feel-good brain hormones. If you suddenly stop taking a high dose of estrogen, you're likely to have a fairly severe withdrawal reaction with hot flashes, night sweats, and extreme mood swings. To avoid a withdrawal reaction, it's best to consult your doctor about very gradually reducing the dose over a period of four to six months.

Once you get the estrogen down to, say, one quarter or one eighth of what you're taking now, you and your physician can decide whether to continue on with some estradiol (a natural estrogen) or use a phytoestrogen such as the red clover extract. You might also want to consider getting a saliva hormone level test at that time to determine whether your estrogen level falls within the ideal range for your age. If not, and the phytoestrogens or progesterone alone are not helping with symptoms, it would be worthwhile to consider supplementation with a low dose of bioidentical estrogen.

Letter from a Reader:
Irritable Bowel Syndrome Clears Up

Dear Dr. Lee,

I am a 59-year-old female, in good health, with the exception of a history of irritable bowel syndrome, with bouts of intestinal cramping and diarrhea, controlled only by taking one Imodium AD daily. My internal medicine specialist recommended *What Your Doctor May* Not *Tell You About Menopause.* He wanted to take me off the pharmaceutical hormones that I had been taking for 20 years, following a total hysterectomy, and to put me on natural hormones compounded specifically for me. I read the book and was so upset I immediately ceased taking the PremPro I had been taking. My doctor tested my hormone levels and compounded natural hormones for me, and I began taking them.

Very slowly, the behavior of my intestines began to change. I found the bouts of cramping and diarrhea slowly diminishing in severity and beginning to be less frequent. I began to wean off the Imodium AD, taking it only when I had to. It took about seven months, but my digestive tract gradually returned to normal. I can eat what I want, when I want, and I no longer have any cramping or diarrhea. The only change I had in my life was stopping the Prempro and taking the natural compounded hormones.

I now feel so much better, more normal, and my moods are better. Your book and my doctor have made a marked difference in my life. Thank you again for your wealth of information, and the new life I have.

From L.W., a grateful reader

How and When to Use Estrogen

Estrogens are controversial hormones because while they have beneficial effects, they can also be deadly if not in balance.

On the plus side, estrogen is responsible for the changes that take place at puberty in girls, such as growth and development of the vagina, uterus, and fallopian tubes. Estrogen causes enlargement of the breasts, contributes to how fat is distributed on the female body, and is involved in bone growth.

In adult women, estrogen contributes to the softness of skin and to vaginal lubrication, helps maintain bone density, and plays an important role in brain function. And of course, estrogen is essential to maintaining a woman's monthly menstrual cycles and the process of conception and pregnancy.

When estrogen is out of balance with the rest of a woman's hormones, it can stimulate out-of-control cell growth, or cancer. It can also cause bloating (water retention), weight gain, and breast tenderness. You'll find a complete list of estrogen's effects on pages 76–77.

Estrone, estradiol, and *estriol* are the three major estrogens made by your body; thus they are natural estrogens. These hormones give you breasts, hips, menstruation, and soft skin, and they play important roles in healthy bones and a healthy heart.

Phytoestrogen is another word for plant estrogen. Phytoestrogens are different from your own estrogens and have a much weaker estrogen effect. Some women are able to successfully treat their menopausal symptoms with phytoestrogens alone. Some examples of plants that contain phytoestrogens are soy and red clover.

Xenoestrogen is another word for a foreign, man-made estrogen that has toxic estrogen effects on the human body. Xenoestrogens are found in most pesticides, plastics, acetones (e.g., nail polish remover), and in industrial pollutants such as PCBs. They can be very potent and toxic, and unlike natural hormones, they aren't efficiently cleared from the body, so they tend to accumulate in tissues.

Equilin is another name for horse estrogen, which is found in Premarin.

Estrogen Dominance and the Danger Zone

Estrogen works safely and effectively in the body when it is present in normal amounts and is balanced by progesterone. When it's not balanced by progesterone, you can have symptoms of *estrogen dominance*. Even if your estrogen levels are normal or low, if you don't have progesterone there to balance it, it can be dangerous.

Symptoms That Can Be Caused or Made Worse by Estrogen Dominance

Acceleration of the aging process

Allergies

Anxiety

Autoimmune disorders such as lupus erythematosus and thyroiditis and possibly Sjögren's disease

Breast tenderness

Breast cancer

Decreased sex drive

Depression

Fat gain, especially around the abdomen, hips, and thighs

Fatigue

Fibrocystic breasts

Foggy thinking

Gallbladder disease

Hair loss

Headaches

Hypoglycemia
Increased blood clotting (increasing risk of strokes)
Infertility
Insomnia (inability to sleep)
Irritability
Memory loss
Migraines (especially premenstrually)
Miscarriage
Osteoporosis
Premenopausal bone loss
PMS
Seizures (related to menstruation)
Strokes
Thyroid dysfunction mimicking hypothyroidism
Uterine cancer
Uterine fibroids
Water retention, bloating

Symptoms of Estrogen Deficiency

Vaginal dryness
Painful intercourse
Urinary tract irritation and/or infection
Hot flashes
Night sweats
Foggy thinking
Fatigue

How Estrogen and Progesterone Balance Each Other

How progesterone balances the unwanted effects of estrogen:

Estrogen Effects	Progesterone Effects
Creates proliferative endometrium	Maintains secretory endometrium
Breast cell stimulation (lumpy or fibrocystic breasts)	Protects against breast fibrocysts
Increased body fat and weight gain	Helps use fat for energy
Salt and fluid retention	Natural diuretic
Depression, anxiety, and headaches	Natural antidepressant and calms anxiety
Cyclical migraines	Prevents cyclical migraines
Poor sleep patterns	Promotes normal sleep patterns
Interferes with thyroid hormone function	Facilitates thyroid hormone function
Impairs blood sugar control	Helps normalize blood sugar levels
Increased risk of blood clots	Normalizes blood clotting
Little or no libido effect	Helps restore normal libido
Loss of zinc and retention of copper	Normalizes zinc and copper levels

Estrogen Effects	Progesterone Effects
Reduced oxygen levels in all cells	Restores proper cell oxygen levels
Causes endometrial cancer	Prevents endometrial cancer
Increased risk of breast cancer	Helps prevent breast cancer
Increased risk of prostate cancer	Decreased risk of prostate cancer
Restrains bone loss	Stimulates new bone formation
Reduces vascular tone (dilates blood vessels)	Improves vascular tone
Triggers autoimmune diseases	Prevents autoimmune diseases
Creates progesterone receptors	Increases sensitivity of estrogen receptors
Relieves hot flashes	Necessary for survival of embryo
Prevents vaginal dryness and mucosal atrophy	Precursor of corticosteroid biosynthesis
Increases risk of gallbladder disease	Prevents coronary artery spasm and atherosclerotic plaque
Improves memory	
Increases brain cell excitability and may cause panic attacks	Improves sleep disorders
Estrogens, especially estriol, improve health of urinary tract	Digestive problems
Relieves night sweats	

Finding the Right Dose of Estrogen for *You*

Estrogen is legally available only by prescription, so you will need to get it from your doctor, who may have his or her own opinions about estrogen dosages and timing. However, many doctors are unfamiliar with the protocols of using natural hormones, and if that is the case, the following information may be helpful.

The best generic answer to the question "What's the right dose of estrogen?" is "the lowest dose possible that will relieve symptoms." What follows is more specific advice, but keep in mind that this information is a starting point. From the beginning you will want to track your symptoms and saliva hormone levels until you find the optimal dose. Be aware that your optimal dose could change. As you age, if you gain or lose weight, substantially change your diet, or start taking other hormones or medications, your need for estrogen can increase or decrease.

There are three major estrogens made by the human body: estriol, estradiol, and estrone.

Estriol has great benefit to the cells of the vagina, but has little effect on breasts or the uterine lining when used conservatively. The good news is that it doesn't seem to promote breast cancer and may even be protective against it. The bad news is that it doesn't help retain bone as well as its more potent sister estrogen, estradiol. However, if a woman has vaginal dryness and/or vaginal cell atrophy, estriol is the best and safest estrogen to use. The recommended dose is just 0.5 mg twice weekly in a cream, applied vaginally. This dose has been used extensively in Western Europe for many years. Used orally, in pill form, it is usually found in combination with estradiol (often called bi-est) in a 1.5 mg dose.

Estradiol is the most widely used and recommended estrogen for menopausal symptoms in general. In the United States, the lowest available dose of oral estradiol (as Estrace, for example) is 0.5 mg. But that tablet is scored, so it will easily break into two halves, each containing 0.25 mg of estradiol. Thus, a bottle of a hundred tablets of 0.5 mg estradiol will last for 200 doses. At 25 doses a month (you'll be taking it every day, with a four- to five-day break each month), that bottle will last for eight months.

Estradiol is also commonly used in patches. They used to be way too heavily dosed, but with the realization that transdermally delivered estradiol is 10 to 20 times more efficient than oral estradiol doses, the amount released has been reduced. The patches available in the United States release 0.1 or 0.025 mg per 24 hours. For most menopausal women the optimal dose will be the 0.025 mg patch.

Estrone is rarely used in natural hormone replacement therapy and we don't recommend it. It is a potent estrogen that is quickly converted to other estrogens and by-products.

Estrogen in a Nutshell

General Guidelines

▶ In general, use the lowest dose possible that relieves symptoms.

▶ Take a four- to five-day break each month.

▶ Track symptoms and get saliva tests to monitor levels.

▶ Apply creams and gels on areas where the skin is thin, such as the palms, inner arms, behind the knees, or in the case of vaginal dryness, apply vaginally. Application is *not* recommended on the face, neck, or breasts. Applying it to fatty areas may slow absorption. Patches work well on upper arms and back.

Dosages

▶ Estradiol (pill): Start with 0.5 or 0.25 mg daily

▶ Estradiol (cream, gel, patch): Start with 0.025 mg daily

▶ Estriol (pill): Start with 1.5 mg daily (usually combined with estradiol)

▶ Estriol (cream, gel): For vaginal dryness, start with 0.5 mg twice weekly

Timing

It is wise to take a little vacation from progesterone and the higher-dose estrogens for four to five days or so each calendar month. Women who are using the low-dose estradiol patch can probably safely do so without the break, as long as their saliva tests show normal levels. Many women find it easiest to remember if they take the break for the first four to five days of each new month. The break helps to re-energize the hormone receptors and it helps to prove that your estrogen doses are not too high. If postmenopausal women take more estrogen than they need, they will have vaginal bleeding (assuming the presence of a uterus) and this will show during the days of not using the hormones. If that happens, reduce the estrogen dose. *There is no reason for postmenopausal women to have periods.* Menstruating past the age of menopause is not going to make you look or feel younger, nor will it slow the aging process.

Should I Use Estrogen Patches or Creams?

One of the issues up on the radar screen in natural hormone replacement therapy is whether oral (pill form) or transdermal (skin cream or patches) works best. A few studies have been published showing that oral estrogen increases levels of C-reactive protein (CRP), a marker of inflammation that is associated with heart disease. Oral estrogens have also been shown in some studies to be associated with dementia and urinary incontinence.

Jane Murray, M.D., who specializes in natural hormone replacement therapy in her medical practice in Kansas City, decided to test this for herself after she noticed that her patients who used estradiol patches seemed to be doing better than those taking pills. She first tested an elderly patient who had been on a small dose of Premarin for many years. When her blood tests showed high CRP levels, Dr. Murray suggested she switch to a patch. After three months on the patch, the patient was tested again, and her CRP levels were normal. According to Dr. Murray, "That was my index case that woke me up to the fact that this is a real and clinically relevant phenomenon. Since then I've had other patients with the same result, so I now routinely recommend patches or cream over pills. I have noticed that my overweight patients who are insulin resistant are more sensitive to the CRP-elevating effects of oral estrogen. This may be why we've gotten such conflicting reports over the years about estrogen's effects on heart disease."

Dr. Murray continues, "I also found that patients on oral hormones tended to have more problems with low libido or sex drive. When I researched this I found that oral hormones stimulate the liver to make proteins, including SBHG [serum binding hormone globulin], which binds to hormones and makes them inactive. When I tested hormone levels in my patients I found that when they were put on oral hormones their SBHG went way up and their free testosterone went way down, which accounts for the low libido. I found this to be true with oral hormone replacement hormones and with birth control pills. When I switched these women to the birth control patches their libido came back."

C. W. (Randy) Randolph, M.D., of Jacksonville Beach, Florida, has had similar results in his busy natural hormone therapy practice, and adds that compared to transdermal estrogens, oral estrogens increase the risk of thromboembolic events (strokes and blood clots). He points out that the liver proteins created by oral estrogens also raise blood pressure, raise triglyceride levels, and suppress thyroid function.

The verdict in a nutshell? Use estrogen patches or creams.

As with progesterone, estrogen creams should be applied in areas where the skin is thin, such as the palms, inner arms, and back of the knees. If you're experiencing vaginal dryness you can apply a small amount there, but check this with your doctor first. According to Dr. David Zava, estrogen creams can have some local effects, so you want to avoid putting it on the breasts, neck, and face.

Although there are commercially available estrogen patches that work well, as of now, there are no commercial brands of estrogen creams or gels, which means only a compounding pharmacist can make them. Most doctors who use natural hormones prefer to work with a compounding pharmacist because from month to month, dosages can be easily adjusted for individual needs.

Estrogen Q&A

Q: Can I get estrogen in an over-the-counter cream or on the Web?

A: You can, but we don't recommend it because estrogen is a prescription-only item and therefore selling it without a prescription is illegal. It's usually safe to assume that companies that will do one thing illegally will do other things illegally. If your estrogen is obtained through a doctor and pharmacist, you have a better chance of safely getting what you need.

Q: Why does my doctor refer to estrogen as E2?

A: In biochemistry, estrone is referred to as E1, estradiol as E2, and estriol as E3. Estradiol is the natural estrogen most often used in HRT.

Q: What are Bi-est and Tri-est?

A: They are natural estrogen creams first created by Jonathan Wright, M.D., that contain a mixture of estrogens in the approximate proportion they are found in your body. Bi-est contains estradiol and estriol, and tri-est contains estradiol, estriol, and estrone. Your doctor can prescribe them for you at a compounding pharmacy.

Q: Both the Women's Health Initiative study and the Million Women Study seem to be saying that the combination of estrogen and a progestin increase the risk of breast cancer, heart attacks, etc., but that estrogen alone isn't a problem. This seems to contradict what you've said about estrogen causing cancer.

A: It's not estrogen by itself that causes breast cancer—most premenopausal women's ovaries make estrogen every month and it doesn't cause cancer. It's excessive doses of estrogen, synthetic estrogens, and estrogen dominance (i.e., no progesterone to balance it) that can increase cancer and stroke risk in particular. A dozen or so other risk factors such as high night cortisol and high insulin levels can contribute to estrogen's cancer-causing effects.

In the Million Women Study, women taking estrogen-only still had a 30 percent increased risk of breast cancer. The Puget Sound Study (Chen, CL et al., *JAMA* 2002; 287:734–741) found that estrogen replacement therapy (estrogen only) increased one's risk of breast cancer (compared to women who never used ERT or HRT) by about 60 percent. Complicating the picture is the fact that we can assume virtually all of the women given estrogen alone have had a hysterectomy, since it well known that estrogen given alone creates a high risk of endometrial (uterine) cancer.

Q: My doctor says that since I've had a hysterectomy and don't have a uterus, I can use estrogen alone.

A: This is an outdated approach to hormone replacement therapy. It came about because back in the 1960s, research revealed that giving estrogen alone sharply increased the risk of endometrial (uterine) cancer. In fact, many thousands of women died of uterine cancer as a result of using estrogen alone. That gave rise to the practice of prescribing a progestin along with the estrogen to protect the uterus. It was assumed that women without a uterus didn't need the progestin, but that was because the research hadn't been done long term to assess the risk of breast cancer and stroke in women who took estrogen alone.

Q: How do you recommend the addition of estrogen to progesterone? Do you take it daily too, and with the same four- to five-day break each month?

A: Yes, if you're postmenopausal you can take estrogen daily with the same four- to five-day break. The key is to keep the dose as low as possible and deliver it in a physio-logical manner, meaning in a way that your body can use it efficiently and effectively. With a low dose patch, you can skip the break. If you're premenopausal, and thus still hav-ing periods, by definition your ovaries are still making es-trogen and you don't need to take supplemental estrogen.

However, women in perimenopause, whose periods may be irregular and whose hormones are fluctuating, may have sporadic low estrogen levels followed by high levels. In this case, if progesterone cream hasn't alleviated symptoms such as hot flashes and night sweats, the mild phytoestrogens such as red clover extract (Promensil, for example) may be effective.

Grapefruit Juice Increases Estrogen Levels

Grapefruit juice slows down the action of the P450 pathways in the liver, meaning that substances cleared from the body through those pathways are held in the body longer. This effect is used to advantage with organ transplant recipients who take their antirejection drugs with grapefruit juice in order to prolong the effects of the drugs.

Estrogen is cleared through similar P450 pathways, and researchers sought to determine whether drinking grapefruit juice with oral (by mouth) estrogen and progesterone would increase hormone levels (Fingerova et al., *Cheska Gynekol,* 2003). Eight healthy postmenopausal volunteers were given 2 mg of oral estradiol valerate and 100 mg of oral micronized progesterone. Blood samples were collected at 0, 2, 3, 5, and 24 hours after the hormones were taken. Serum levels of estradiol and progesterone were measured by radio immune assay (RIA). The same trial was repeated a week later but the hormone pills were swallowed with 200 ml of grapefruit juice. Grapefruit juice on average slightly increased serum levels of estradiol and progesterone; this increase reached statistical significance only for the estradiol level 24 hours after the hormones were taken. The variability of response to the progesterone was so great that the researchers were unable to draw a conclusion.

These researchers would have had a lot more information to work with if they had used saliva hormone levels, which measure bioavailable hormones. Oral progesterone is broken down into many metabolites as it moves through the digestive system, and this may account for the variability of results.

While this chapter gives you specific instructions on the dosage and timing of estrogen use, it is important to work with your doctor to track your symptoms and hormone levels. *And remember, even if you have had a hysterectomy, you should never use estrogen without progesterone to accompany it.* In the next chapter, we'll move on to testosterone, a hormone that's important to women as well as men.

How and When to Use Testosterone

Testosterone is an *androgen,* or male hormone, but women also make it in small amounts. In women, testosterone primarily contributes to sex drive, or libido, and helps build bone. It can increase energy and improve the ability to focus on a task such as balancing the checkbook. Testosterone has also been shown to improve symptoms such as vaginal dryness, incontinence, and urinary tract problems, but this may be due to the fact that in women, much of it is converted to estrogen.

Testosterone deficiency can cause loss of energy, depression, memory lapses, bone loss, and loss of libido. Similar symptoms can also be caused by adrenal exhaustion or thyroid deficiency, so it's wise to have your doctor check these possibilities or test testosterone levels before supplementing it.

Women with an excess of testosterone often have symptoms of hair loss on the head, excessive hair growth on the rest of the body, acne, polycystic ovary syndrome (PCOS), and irritability or "testiness."

PCOS is most often caused by a poor diet that is heavy on sugar and refined carbohydrates, and light on fruits, vegetables, and whole grains, along with lack of exercise. This type of lifestyle can create chronically high insulin levels, which stimulate the production of testosterone by the ovaries, which can lead to ovarian cysts. PCOS can be a painful and debilitating problem, and yet can be resolved in most women within a few months with a strict change in diet and an increase in exercise. Please read *What Your Doctor May* Not *Tell You About Premenopause* for details.

After menopause, usually when a woman is in her early to mid-fifties, the ovaries produce about 60 percent less estrogen and almost no progesterone, but often continue producing a small amount of testosterone well into the seventies. As a result, testosterone supplementation is often not needed in a menopausal woman.

When to Use Testosterone

If you have used progesterone cream for at least six months (see chapter 9 for details) and still have a low libido, check your testosterone and DHEA levels to see if the problem could be due to low androgens (male hormones). Sometimes lack of sex drive is caused by other hormonal imbalances such as low thyroid or high stress hormones like cortisol. In testing saliva and monitoring symptoms, Dr. David Zava of ZRT Laboratory has seen many cases where women had perfectly normal, and sometimes high androgen levels, but still suffered from low libido. These women usually had other problems such as high stress and symptoms of low thyroid caused by estrogen dominance. Excessive estrogen or excessive natural progesterone replacement therapy can also suppress libido, so if you are taking these hormones check the levels of estradiol and progesterone to make sure you are not using too much.

Dr. Zava has found with saliva testing that the majority of women who have had their ovaries removed along with hysterectomy suffer from low androgens (testosterone, DHEA-S, and androstenedione). A recent study found that after "complete" hysterectomy (i.e., ovaries removed) women often suffer low energy, depression, and lack of libido. Testing "free" testosterone (not the usual serum testing) showed that these women were testosterone deficient. Transdermal testosterone, in doses of 0.15 mg/day, raised their "free" testosterone levels five-fold and effectively relieved their symptoms. Clinicians report that they successfully use transdermal doses (creams, gels) of 0.15 to 1 mg per day, with the average dose for a menopausal woman being 0.5 mg daily.

Testosterone is available in the form of cream, sublingual drops, oral tablets, and transdermal patch. A compounding pharmacist can formulate testosterone creams and sublingual drops. Combining testosterone and progesterone into one cream is not recommended. It's so easy for a woman to get too much testosterone that you need to be able to adjust your dosage if you notice symptoms of excess.

Testosterone is available only by prescription. If you're interested, talk with your physician. Be sure to use only a natural form, because synthetics like methyltestosterone are powerful and can have unpleasant side effects. Estratest contains methyltestosterone and is not recommended.

Dr. David Zava has found that for some women, particularly those who have had their ovaries surgically removed, both DHEA and testosterone are low. In these cases, supplementing with DHEA may raise both DHEA and testosterone levels. In this case, a low dose of DHEA—5 to 10 mg daily—can be a good alternative to testosterone supplementation since it's available over the counter and is less expensive. Some women, however, readily convert DHEA to estrogen, so saliva testing is recommended before and after starting DHEA supplements.

9

The ABCs of Progesterone

Progesterone is the hormone that's most often out of balance or deficient in women. Supplementing with natural progesterone cream in the right timing and dosage can often quickly and effectively solve the majority of hormone imbalances. If you're interested in delving into the myriad of reasons for this twenty-first-century phenomenon, please read *What Your Doctor May Not Tell You About Menopause,* or *What Your Doctor May Not Tell You About Premenopause.*

In this chapter you'll find some basic questions and answers about progesterone that will help you decide whether to use it.

What Is Progesterone?

Progesterone is a steroid hormone made by the ovaries when you ovulate (release an egg) in the middle of your menstrual cycle. It's also made in smaller amounts by the adrenal glands, and in even smaller amounts by some nerve cells. Progesterone is manufactured in the body from a steroid hormone called pregnenolone and is a precursor to most of the other steroid hormones, including cortisol, androstenedione, the estrogens, and testosterone, meaning that the body manufactures most of the other steroid hormones from progesterone. However, if you use supplemental progesterone, it will not raise your levels of the other hormones—that conversion apparently takes place prior to progesterone's arrival in the bloodstream.

A woman with normal menstrual cycles produces 20 to 30 mg of progesterone daily from the middle to the end of her menstrual cycle. That's why the goal in hormone replacement is to use that dose of progesterone.

Menstrual Cycle

One Normal Cycle = 18 to 32 days

Period Day 1_____→ _____Ovulation_____→ _____Period Day 1

| Estrogen rising | Progesterone rising | Estrogen and progesterone falling |

Progesterone's most important role is to balance or oppose the effects of estrogen. By itself, estrogen creates a strong risk for breast cancer and reproductive cancers, as well as a long list of other symptoms (see chapter 7 for details). Progesterone also stimulates bone building and thus helps protect against osteoporosis. (Estrogen also plays an important role in bone health by slowing bone loss.)

Estrogen levels drop only about 60 percent at menopause, which is just enough to stop the menstrual cycle. But progesterone levels may drop to near zero in some women.

Progestin Versus Progesterone

Progesterone is preferable to the synthetic progestins such as Provera, because it is natural to the body and has virtually no undesirable side effects when used as directed.

If you have any doubts about how different progesterone is from the progestins, in the third trimester of pregnancy, the placenta produces 300 to 400 mg of progesterone daily, so we know that such levels are safe for a developing baby. But progestins, even at fractions of this dose, can cause birth defects.

The Women's Health Initiative found that the combination of estrogen and a progestin in HRT caused a significantly higher risk of breast cancer, strokes, and heart disease, while a 10-year French study of estrogen and progesterone found no negative side effects.

The progestins can also cause many other health problems, including partial loss of vision, fluid retention, migraine headaches, asthma, and depression. To appreciate the scope of progestin side effects, it is instructive to review the *Physicians' Desk Reference (PDR)* pages for medroxyprogesterone acetate. An *abbreviated* list from the *Physicians' Desk Reference (PDR)* follows.

Potential Side Effects of Medroxyprogesterone Acetate (Provera)

Warning for Women
There is an increased risk of minor birth defects in children whose mothers take this drug during the first four months of pregnancy. [Genital abnormalities, which the children might not consider "minor."]

Warnings
    Beagle dogs given this drug developed mammary nodules, some of which were malignant.

    The physician should be alert to the earliest manifestation of thrombotic disorders (thrombophlebitis, cerebrovascular disorders, pulmonary embolism, and retinal thrombosis).

Discontinue this drug if there is sudden partial or complete loss of vision.

Detectable amounts of progestin have been identified in the milk of mothers receiving the drug. The effect of this on the nursing neonate and infant has not been determined.

Contraindications

Thrombophlebitis, thromboembolic disorders, cerebral apoplexy; liver dysfunction or disease; known or suspected malignancy of breast or genital organs; undiagnosed vaginal bleeding; missed abortion; known or suspected pregnancy.

Precautions

Because progestogens may cause some degree of fluid retention, conditions which might be influenced by this factor, such as epilepsy, migraine, asthma, cardiac or renal dysfunction, require careful observation.

May cause breakthrough bleeding or menstrual irregularities.

May cause or contribute to depression.

The effect of prolonged use of this drug on pituitary, ovarian, adrenal, hepatic, or uterine function is unknown.

May decrease glucose tolerance; diabetic patients must be carefully monitored.

May increase the thrombotic disorders associated
with estrogens.

Adverse Reactions

Breast tenderness and galactorrhea.

Sensitivity reactions such as urticaria, pruritus,
edema, or rash.

Acne, alopecia, and hirsutism (excess hair growth).

Edema, weight changes (increase or decrease).

Cervical erosions and changes in cervical secretions.

Cholestatic jaundice.

Mental depression, pyrexia, nausea, insomnia, or
somnolence.

Anaphylactoid reactions and anaphylaxis (severe
acute allergic reactions).

Thrombophlebitis and pulmonary embolism.

Breakthrough bleeding, spotting, amenorrhea, or
changes in menses.

Fatigue, backache, itching, dizziness, nervousness,
loss of scalp hair.

When Taken with Estrogens, the Following Have Been Observed

Rise in blood pressure, headache, dizziness,
nervousness, fatigue.

Changes in sex drive, hirsutism and loss of scalp hair,
decrease in T3 uptake values.

Premenstrual-like syndrome, changes in appetite.

Cystitis-like syndrome (urinary tract infections).

Erythema multiforme, erythema nodosum, hemor-
rhagic eruption, itching.

Estrogen Dominance

Dr. Lee coined the term "estrogen dominance" to describe
what happens when the normal ratio or balance of estrogen to progesterone is changed by excess estrogen or
inadequate progesterone. Estrogen is a potent and potentially dangerous hormone when not balanced by adequate progesterone.

Women who have suffered from both PMS and menopausal symptoms will recognize the hallmark symptoms
of estrogen dominance: weight gain, bloating, mood
swings, irritability, tender breasts, headaches, fatigue, depression, hypoglycemia, uterine fibroids, endometriosis,
and fibrocystic breasts. Estrogen dominance is known to
cause and/or contribute to cancer of the breast, ovary, en-
dometrium (uterus), and prostate (in men).

In the 10 to 15 years before menopause, many
women regularly have anovulatory (no ovulation) cycles
in which they make enough estrogen to create menstruation, but they don't make any progesterone, thus setting
the stage for estrogen dominance. Using progesterone

cream during anovulatory months can help prevent the symptoms of PMS. You'll know when you're having an anovulatory month if you start to get PMS or estrogen dominance symptoms around the middle of your cycle.

PMS can occur despite normal progesterone levels when stress is present. Stress increases production of the hormone cortisol, which blocks (or competes for) progesterone receptors. That means progesterone won't work. Additional progesterone is required to overcome this blockade, and stress management is important.

What Is Progesterone Made From?

The progesterone used for hormone replacement comes from plant fats and oils, usually a substance called diosgenin that is extracted from a very specific type of wild yam that grows in Mexico, or from soybeans. These days, virtually all progesterone is made from soybeans. In the laboratory, diosgenin is chemically synthesized into a molecular structure that is identical to real human progesterone. The other human steroid hormones, including estrogen, testosterone, progesterone, and the cortisones are also nearly always synthesized from diosgenin.

Some companies try to sell diosgenin, which they label "wild yam extract" as a medicine or supplement, claiming that the body will then convert it into hormones as needed. While we know this can be done in the laboratory, this conversion does *not* take place in the human body. That's why we recommend not using progesterone creams labeled "wild yam" unless you know for sure that they contain the proper amount of real progesterone.

How to Use Progesterone

Sometimes using progesterone cream really is as easy as following the instructions on the jar or bottle, but if not, there's a good chance you can find answers to your "how to" questions in this chapter. Having said this, it's always preferable to work in partnership with a skilled and competent health care professional when balancing your hormones. It is notoriously difficult to be objective in diagnosing and treating oneself, and tracking whatever changes might be taking place. With or without a health care professional to work with, it's a great idea, at least for the first few months of beginning a hormone balance regimen, to keep a daily journal that records what you ate, what you took in the way of supplements, and how you feel.

Creams, Drops, Pills, or Suppositories?

Creative health professionals have come up with all sorts of ways to take supplemental progesterone. You can put it in the orifice of your choice: oral, vaginal, rectal, or nasal. You can inject it, insert it, spray it, swallow it, suck on it, or rub it in. The only form that progesterone doesn't come in at this time is a patch, but don't be surprised if that's available soon.

In choosing the delivery method, let's consider both convenience and what most closely approximates what your body would do.

Convenience would eliminate vaginal and rectal applications because they're messy and leaky. Crinone is an example of a vaginal progesterone.

Injections are out because they involve alcohol swabs, needles, and soreness at the injection site.

Nasal sprays are a fairly efficient delivery method but the jury is out on the long-term effects of delivering progesterone directly to the brain (which is what happens, at least in part, when you spray it up your nose), and they reportedly taste terrible.

If you suck on a lozenge or put drops under your tongue, you'll get a steep, sudden rise in progesterone levels, followed by a steep drop, which doesn't mimic what your body would do. The rapid rise and fall of progesterone leaves you without progesterone for a good part of the day unless you take it every few hours—that's inconvenient.

If you take a pill, as much as 95 percent of the progesterone will be converted to inactive by-products in the gastrointestinal tract before it ever gets to the bloodstream, so you have to take 100 mg to get 5 mg into the bloodstream. Prometrium is an example of a commercially available progesterone pill where typical doses range from 100 to 300 mg.

Delivering a substance to the body through the skin is known as a *transdermal* application. Transdermal progesterone—cream, gel, and oil—is absorbed through the skin into the underlying fat layer, from which it diffuses into the capillaries permeating the fat, where it can be taken up slowly in the blood. It begins circulating in the blood within seconds of application and reaches its peak in about 3 to 4 hours. Levels then drop rapidly for 8 to 12 hours, and steadily for 12 to 24 hours, reaching baseline (before progesterone) in 12 to 36 hours. This is why it works best to use progesterone cream twice daily to most closely mimic how your body functions. Clearly, transdermal application is the most convenient and effective form of supplemental progesterone.

The question of whether topical or transdermal progesterone is well absorbed isn't even debatable anymore. It's been repeatedly proven in a variety of good, published studies to be efficiently absorbed into the bloodstream, from where it's well dispersed into the rest of the tissues in the body. The fact that conventional medicine is now delivering all manner of hormones via patches at much lower doses than oral forms should be a good indicator that hormones can be effectively absorbed through the skin. In fact, of all the steroid hormones, progesterone is the most easily absorbed. If you'd like the details of these studies and the biochemistry behind them, please read *What Your Doctor May Not Tell You About Menopause* or *What Your Doctor May Not Tell You About Premenopause.*

There are those who claim that transdermal progesterone overaccumulates in the fat cells and creates extremely high levels of progesterone in the body. This can happen if you take too much progesterone, but otherwise it's rare. Normally progesterone moves from fat cells into the bloodstream and to tissues of the body as needed.

Applying Progesterone Cream

Transdermal progesterone cream is very easily and quickly absorbed into the body, so you can apply it almost anywhere with success. However, it's wise to rotate the areas to which you apply it, to avoid saturating any one area. It is best absorbed where the skin is relatively thin and well supplied with capillary blood flow, such as the face, neck, upper chest, breasts, inner arms, and the palms of the hands and soles of the feet.

Women differ in almost every aspect of their physiology. Although genetically all humans are 99 percent the same, that 1 percent difference can account for an astounding variation in how the details work. It's not rational for a doctor to order the same dose of any given medicine for every patient, and the same is true of natural progesterone.

While medical professionals can give you guidelines to work within, it's up to you to find the best dose for your body. Ideally, you should be able to find the minimum amount you can use to gain and sustain relief from your symptoms. Because natural progesterone is so safe, it won't hurt you to use a little more than your optimal dose. That gives you plenty of room for experimentation. You'll find specific recommendations in chapter 10.

As with most substances, too much progesterone will cause problems. As the use of progesterone has increased in popularity, health care professionals have developed many different schools of thought about how to use it, and many of them prescribe very high doses of progesterone. This practice is counterproductive and leads to further hormone imbalance, not to mention a handful of interesting theories about why the progesterone isn't working the way Dr. Lee says it does. Here's the answer, folks: it's the overdose!

Chronically high doses of progesterone over many months eventually cause progesterone receptors to turn off, reducing its effectiveness. Using excessive doses of progesterone can also cause the side effects listed below. Not all women suffer from these side effects when they use excessive doses of progesterone, but eventually their symptoms will return.

Symptoms may also return if the underlying causes of your hormonal imbalance haven't been addressed. This could include stress, poor diet, obesity, lack of exercise, lack of sleep, thyroid deficiency, and adrenal fatigue. All of these factors are covered in detail in *What Your Doctor May Not Tell You About Menopause* and *What Your Doctor May Not Tell You About Premenopause*.

Not All "Wild Yam Extract" Is Progesterone

A word of caution: Not all products with labels claiming "wild yam extract" actually contain any progesterone. Some do, some don't. By historical practice, many nutritional products have merely listed their ingredients by such nonspecific labeling. Thus, "wild yam extract" may be ground up wild yam, it may be diosgenin (an extract of wild yam), or it may be progesterone. If progesterone is not specifically listed on the label, the only way to find out if it is included is to call the company. Furthermore, some of these "wild yam creams" contain very small amounts of progesterone, so if the amount of progesterone is not listed on the label or in a brochure, make sure to find out how much it contains. Since there are many excellent progesterone creams available at reasonable prices, the best approach may be to stick with creams that are clearly labeled.

Possible Side Effects of Progesterone

Dr. Lee used to say that there are no known side effects of progesterone when it is taken in small physiologic doses, that is, 20 or so milligrams per day. However, over more than a decade of having millions of people read his books, newsletters, and website, he learned that to make such a blanket statement was to invite mail that informed him to the contrary. The majority of the time these so-called side effects have good reasons to exist. The most common reason for progesterone cream side effects is gross overdose. We have heard tales of health care professionals and pharmacists recommending a 100 mg daily dosage of progesterone cream. This type of medical mismanagement is guaranteed to cause not just side effects, but serious hormonal imbalances, including a shutting down of hormone receptors. Another common cause of side effects are the creams that include a mix of other hormones such as estrogen and testosterone. Transdermal hormones should be taken individually so that you can regulate dosage if you experience symptoms of overdose or deficiency.

Extremely large doses of progesterone can cause sleepiness, although most women report they simply feel calm. Enormous doses can cause an anesthetic or drunken effect.

Some women report estrogen dominance symptoms for a week or two after starting progesterone, but this is caused by a sensitization of estrogen receptors and generally disappears within a few weeks. In some women it may take a few months for hormones to balance out.

If you're still having periods and you take progesterone out of phase with your cycle, it may change the timing of your period or cause some spotting.

Overall, the percentage of women who genuinely suffer from side effects is extremely small and may be due to rare individual variations in biochemistry or some type of autoimmune reaction.

The following is a list of possible progesterone side effects:

Lethargy/sleepiness This is probably an effect of allopregnanolone, a by-product of progesterone, on the brain.

Edema (water retention) This is probably caused by excess conversion to deoxycorticosterone, a mineralocorticoid made in the adrenal glands that causes water retention.

Candida This bacteria is present in a yeast infection; excess progesterone can inhibit anti-candida neutrophils (white blood cells).

Bloating Excess progesterone slows gastrointestinal (GI) transport, and with the wrong kind of gastrointestinal flora such as candida this can lead to bloating and gas. (During pregnancy the high levels of progesterone slow food transport through the GI tract to enhance absorption of nutrients.)

Lowered libido Excessive progesterone may lower one's libido because in very high doses it blocks the conversion of testosterone to its more potent metabolites that play a role in libido.

Mild depression Excess progesterone down-regulates estrogen receptors, and brain response to estrogens is needed for serotonin production.

Exacerbates symptoms of estrogen deficiency Excess progesterone down-regulates estrogen receptors and desensitizes tissue to estrogen. Because progesterone receptors are dependent on estrogen priming through the estrogen receptor, excess progesterone in the absence of estrogen can cause a lot of problems. This can be especially true in women who have very low estradiol and are taking large doses of progesterone.

Progesterone metabolites Then there's the question of progesterone metabolites (some mentioned in the list above), the by-products created by excessive progesterone. In addition to the above-listed side effects, they certainly put an extra and unnecessary burden on the liver as it works overtime to excrete them. This happens most frequently when women use oral progesterone (pill form). As much as 90 percent of an oral dose is destroyed in the gastrointestinal tract within 15 minutes or so of taking it. The progesterone that is destroyed becomes by-products or metabolites that enter the liver, where they and the real progesterone are transported into the bloodstream. Several research groups, including one in France (Nahoul) and another in the United States (Levin), using highly sophisticated methods of analysis, came to the conclusion that about 80 percent of what is measured as progesterone by conventional blood tests is really inactive metabolites of progesterone. Therefore, if you are taking 100 mg of oral progesterone and your blood test comes back as 10 nanograms per milliliter, the real progesterone level is more likely only to be about 2 ng/ml and the rest of it inactive metabolites or metabolites that may cause side effects rather than benefits. These metabolites are not as likely to get into saliva, and therefore a measurement of bioavailable progesterone (through a saliva test) will give far more accurate levels than blood serum (or plasma) levels.

Some doctors prescribe oral progesterone for women who are having trouble sleeping, because one of its side effects is often sleepiness. However, if you're working or driving a vehicle, sleepiness is counterproductive.

Breast Heaviness, Bloating, and Fatigue: It's the Deoxycorticosterone

Very high doses of progesterone over time can convert to a hormone called deoxycorticosterone in *some* women. How much of this hormone is made can vary a great deal from woman to woman and is probably a function of your genetic makeup. If you're predisposed to make a lot of this progesterone by-product, you may suffer from breast heaviness, bloating, and fatigue if your progesterone level is too high. This conversion can also happen in *some* women who are under a great deal of stress over a long period of time.

Too Little Progesterone

While some women take too much progesterone, there are also creams out there with virtually no progesterone in them (5 to 10 mg per jar of cream), and women who use those creams are under-dosed. Ten mg of progesterone per jar of cream is not enough to oppose the effects of estrogen or to build bone. In fact, the very low dose progesterone may make estrogen even more active and make estrogen dominance symptoms worse. These creams are *not* recommended. It's important to know how much progesterone is in the cream you're using.

Will using progesterone cream raise your other hormone levels?

Progesterone does not cause an increase in the levels of other steroid hormones. This is probably because progesterone cream is carried directly through the fat layer in your skin and into the bloodstream, while the conversion of progesterone made in the body into other hormones takes place directly in the ovaries and adrenal glands.

Now that you know the ABCs of progesterone, in the next chapter we'll give you detailed information on how much progesterone to use, and the timing.

10

How and When to Use Progesterone Cream

In this chapter, we'll first give you general information on when to use progesterone cream, then we'll go into dosages and different ways of using it for specific problems. The majority of women who use progesterone cream alone to create hormone balance can simply follow the directions on the container, but if you or your doctor have questions about specific problems, this chapter will assist you in finding the right dosage and timing for your individual needs. The information in this chapter is based on using a two-ounce jar of progesterone cream that contains 900 to 1,000 mg of progesterone.

A progesterone-deficient woman who starts using natural progesterone cream in the recommended doses will find that, in three to four months, the progesterone in her body fat will reach physiologic equilibrium. Most women will be able to judge for themselves, based on symptoms, that the previous hormone imbalance is now corrected.

Apply Once or Twice Daily

Progesterone cream can be applied once or twice a day. If you know you're not going to remember to apply it twice a day, then apply the full dose once a day. The optimal approach is a divided dose, with a larger dose at bedtime and a smaller dose in the morning. Getting each dab of cream to be exactly the right size isn't that important here, because there's a buffering effect as the progesterone is absorbed into subcutaneous (under the skin) fat. The release of the hormone from body fat serves to make the progesterone effect relatively steady even if daily doses vary somewhat.

Doses for Premenopausal Women

Most premenopausal women need only 15 to 20 mg of progesterone daily during the middle phase of their cycle, which is about what the body would make if it was making its own progesterone. Some women have better results using up to 30 mg, and others with closer to 10 mg.

If you are taking a physiologic dose (an amount approximating what your body would make itself under normal circumstances) and your symptoms don't go away after four to six months, or if they return, it's best to work in partnership with a competent health care professional to find out why. In many cases other hormone imbalances need to be corrected, most commonly estrogen deficiency, androgen deficiency (particularly problematic in women who have had a hysterectomy), poor adrenal function causing low or high cortisol levels, or thyroid deficiency. There is almost never a reason to add an estrogen supplement to a woman still having monthly periods; the very fact that she is menstruating is evidence that she is making plenty of estrogen.

> **There is almost never a reason to add an estrogen supplement to a woman still having monthly periods; the very fact that she is menstruating is evidence that she is making plenty of estrogen.**

Menopausal Women and Women Who've Had a Hysterectomy (with or without ovaries)

After menopause, the ovaries continue to make small amounts of estrogen and testosterone. In addition, estrogen continues to be made by body fat. In two-thirds of menopausal women, estradiol levels are sufficient, but progesterone levels may fall to nearly zero.

In a menopausal woman, I have found that 10 to 12 mg of progesterone per day for 24 to 25 days of the calendar month works well. That is ⅛ teaspoonful. A two-ounce container will easily last for at least three months.

A woman with a hysterectomy is in surgically induced menopause and can follow the same instructions. Even if the surgeon spared your ovaries, they are likely to stop functioning within a year or two after a hysterectomy. According to Dr. David Zava, testosterone is nearly always low in a woman who has had a hysterectomy. One way to find out if your ovaries are still functioning is to have a saliva hormone level test before you start using supplemental hormones.

The First Few Months

Ultimately, how you achieve your monthly dosing goal will probably come down to personal preference, and perhaps the personal preference of your health care professional. How you're feeling will be a good indicator of whether it's working for you. In a very few women, the first few weeks of starting a hormone balance regimen can involve some worsening of symptoms and even new ones, but that phase generally passes quickly. If you feel fine for four to six months on a given dose, and then find it is not working as well, this is usually a sign that you should reduce your dose. A saliva test will be helpful here.

If you have been taking too much progesterone, or your saliva levels are out of range, simply cut way back on the dose or go off the cream for a few months.

Why You Want to Avoid High Doses of Progesterone

BY DR. DAVID ZAVA

I would define a higher dose progesterone cream as a product containing 10 percent progesterone and delivered in about a ¼ teaspoon, meaning that total progesterone delivery to the skin is about 100 mg. A lower dose progesterone cream is one containing about 1.5 to 2 percent progesterone, which delivers about 10 to 20 mg of progesterone in ¼ teaspoon of cream.

Women who use higher dose progesterone creams have much higher saliva progesterone levels (saliva levels usually exceed 10,000 pg/ml), and are more likely to have side effects such as bloating, slowed digestion, sleepiness, and mild depression. Some women have exacerbation of candida, both in the digestive tract and as vaginal yeast infections. At a really high dose, progesterone can start converting into DOC or deoxycortico-sterone, which is a mineralocorticoid that in excess can cause water retention and swelling.

Women using the higher dose progesterone creams may

eventually experience symptoms of estrogen deficiency. These are the women who say the cream relieved their symptoms for three months, or a year, but now they've returned. They have pushed their progesterone too far and have developed what I would term progesterone dominance, or lack of balance with estrogens. This can happen even in women on the lower dose creams. Estrogens and progesterone depend on each other for balance. We always think about the need for progesterone to balance estrogen, but progesterone won't work without a little bit of estrogen. For progesterone to be most effective requires a little estrogen priming.

At the cell level, estrogen stimulates cells to make progesterone receptors, which in turn allows cells to respond to progesterone. Progesterone binds to its receptor and the ensuing events result in regulation of estrogen receptors. When the progesterone dose gets high enough, it down-regulates estrogen receptors, shutting off further tissue response to estrogens, particularly estrogen-stimulated cell growth.

How to Get the Most Out of Your Progesterone Cream

Here are some general guidelines on how to get the most out of your progesterone cream dose:

▶ The larger the area of skin the dose is spread on, the greater the absorption.

▶ Apply the cream to thinner skin with high capillary density – such as places where you blush. Through testing at his lab, Dr. David Zava has found that the best spots are the palms (if they aren't callused), chest, inner arms, neck, and face. The soles of the feet are also good if they're not thickened from walking barefoot.

▶ Progesterone cream should be applied after, not before, a warm bath or shower.

▶ If you use the cream at bedtime it can be calming and help you sleep. If you apply it twice a day, use a larger dab at night and a smaller one in the morning.

▶ Since other ingredients of the cream are generally not absorbed, continual use of any single skin area will eventually saturate that area, and this might reduce progesterone absorption. Rotate among three or four different skin sites on different days.

Progesterone Cream Timing and Dosage

Again, please keep in mind that it is not helpful to use too much progesterone cream and that all of the dosage recommendations in this chapter are based on using a two-ounce container of progesterone cream that contains a total of 900 to 1,000 mg of progesterone per two-ounce container, or 450 to 500 mg per ounce (for your compounding pharmacist, this is a 1.6 to 2 percent progesterone cream). This amounts to about 40 mg per ½ teaspoon, 20 mg per ¼ teaspoon, and 10 mg per ⅛ teaspoon.

Menopausal (not having menstrual cycles)

A general guideline is to use a total daily dose of 10 to 20 mg of progesterone cream for 24 to 26 days of the calendar month. If you experience a recurrence of hot flashes or other symptoms during the break you can try reducing the dose gradually over a two- to three-day period before taking the break, or if that doesn't work, reduce the break time to just three days completely off.

> **The use of progesterone cream will not prevent menopause or aging from occurring—but it sure can help with the symptoms!**

It's best to apply the cream in divided doses: half before bed and half in the morning. However, if that doesn't work well for you, don't be concerned. Just pick one time of the day when it's most convenient to apply it and use the whole dose.

Hysterectomy or Ovariectomy

A hysterectomy is, in effect, instant menopause. The difference is that the ovaries of women in normal menopause are making small amounts of estrogens and androgens for many years (often well into the seventies). Women with a "complete" hysterectomy (removal of the uterus and the ovaries) aren't making any hormones at all (except for very small amounts in the adrenal glands).

The abruptness of a complete hysterectomy is hard on the body. If you have had your ovaries surgically removed (ovariectomy or oophorectomy), all the ovarian hormones are lost. Hormone replacement in these circumstances should include low dose estrogen and natural progesterone cream in normal physiological doses for 24 to 26 days of the calendar month. Many women, after removal of their ovaries, also have testosterone deficiency, causing low energy levels, depression, bone loss, and lack of libido. If present, testosterone deficiency can be effectively treated by transdermal testosterone in doses as low as 0.15 mg/day. (See chapter 8 for details on supplemental testosterone.)

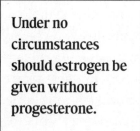

Under no circumstances should estrogen be given without progesterone.

Perimenopausal

Perimenopause is the transition time between pre-menopause and menopause. This can be a time of irregular periods, hot flashes and night sweats, fluctuating libido and emotions, heavy bleeding, and the first real signs of aging. As you approach menopause, estrogen production often becomes more variable. Under such circumstances, it may be unrealistic to expect to have regular cycles, or perfect hormone balance, even with progesterone cream.

It's best to synchronize your natural progesterone supplementation with your body's own hormonal cycles as much as possible. If you're having irregular periods, breakthrough bleeding, or spotting, use your intuition about when to start and stop the cream and be sure to see your doctor if it occurs every few weeks for more than a few months. You may want to try to time it according to when your periods were regular.

The use of progesterone cream will not prevent menopause from occurring.

Premenopausal

Women's sensitivity to hormones differs tremendously, so your dose will depend upon your individual biochemistry.

Use 15 to 30 mg of progesterone during the two weeks prior to your period, stopping a day or two before the expected period. For most women, 20 mg is the optimal dose, but you can experiment to find out what is optimal for you. If you have an average length cycle of 28 to 30 days you can begin using progesterone on day 12 of your cycle, counting the first day of your period as day 1. If your cycle is longer or shorter than 28 to 30 days, you can start two weeks before day 1 of your next period is due (see sidebar on page 129 for details).

Anovulatory Cycles and Luteal Insufficiency

A saliva hormone test that shows low progesterone levels, indicates either that you haven't ovulated (an anovulatory cycle) or that you are unable to produce the proper amount of progesterone after ovulation (luteal insufficiency). Both are quite common among women between the ages of 35 and 50 and are often the cause of PMS, infertility, and miscarriages. In one study (Prior, JC, et al., *Lancet*, 1992) on a group of 18 regularly cycling women, with an average age of 29, seven of them (39 percent) were found to be anovulatory and were not producing progesterone.

Dr. David Zava finds with saliva testing that anovulation is usually associated with both low estradiol and low progesterone, and occurs frequently in women who have been on birth control, particularly Depo-Provera. These women often suffer with symptoms characteristic of both

Even when I ovulate, confirmed with a test, I still have have estrogen dominance symptoms the last two weeks of my cycle.

Even if you can tell that you have ovulated, it does not mean that you do not need progesterone supplementation. Ovulation does not guarantee continued progesterone production during the last two weeks of your cycle. In many women, progesterone production may fall shortly after ovulation and they become estrogen dominant again in the week before their period. This is called luteal phase failure, and it is common in U.S. women after age 35. Luteal phase failure is a common cause of irregular cycles and infertility.

estrogen and progesterone deficiency. Luteal insufficiency is associated with normal to high estrogen and low progesterone, along with a host of estrogen dominance symptoms. Luteal insufficiency may also be associated with the use of other forms of chemical birth control such as pills and patches.

Some Women Need a Loading Dose
A loading dose is a higher-than-normal dose taken to quickly raise hormone levels back to normal. This can be

useful for women who have had many months or years of anovulatory cycles, creating extreme progesterone deficiency. Each anovulatory cycle sends a woman deeper into estrogen dominance as body fat progesterone stores are depleted. Very thin women with little body fat go into estrogen dominance much more quickly. In such women, the first one or two months of transdermal progesterone are used to replenish body fat stores, so it makes sense to use higher doses during that time. After two to three months of progesterone use, the dose can usually be reduced with good effect. Women who start out using ¼ teaspoon of cream twice a day (40 mg/day) for the two weeks prior to their period usually find that they can reduce the dose by half (20 mg/day) for these same two weeks each month and continue to have good results.

We can't emphasize enough that the bottom line in progesterone dosing is always observing and tracking symptoms. Have your PMS symptoms improved? Are you gaining less weight before your periods? Are your breast or uterine cysts getting smaller? Are your moods steadier? Are you less anxious? It's all about working to find the dose that corrects the problem, then reducing that dose to the minimum needed to maintain the desired effect. However, if you're using more than 50 mg of progesterone daily for more than a few months, there's something other than a progesterone deficiency that's wrong, and it's important to delve deeper and work with your doctor to find out what it is.

The Best Way to Calculate When to Use Progesterone Cream if You're Having Periods

Day 1 of your cycle is the first day of your period. The conventional wisdom is that a menstrual cycle lasts 28 days, and that ovulation occurs at mid-cycle, or at day 12 to 14. Women who have 28-day cycles will usually do fine starting progesterone on the twelfth to fourteenth day of their cycle. But how about women with shorter or longer cycles? A normal menstrual cycle can last anywhere from 18 to 32 days. If you start using progesterone cream on the twelfth day of an 18- or 32-day cycle, you're likely to start having symptoms such as breakthrough bleeding and irregular periods.

Here's what you do: Get out a calendar and figure out when day 1 of your next period is due, based on a normal cycle *for you*. Then count backward two weeks, and that's when you would start using the progesterone.

Why does this work so well? Because the number of days between day 1 of your period and when ovulation begins can vary quite a lot from woman to woman, but the number of days between ovulation and day 1 of the period is consistently two weeks.

Menstrual Cycle

Period Day 1____ → ____Ovulation____ → ____Period Day 1

# of days varies   2 weeks

Endometriosis

Women with endometriosis have small bits of endometrial (uterine) tissue scattered here and there about the uterus, other pelvic organs, the wall of the colon, and even in the lungs. While the cause is not clear, these islets of endometrial tissue respond to estrogen just as the endometrial cells in the uterus do—they fill with blood each month and can cause severe pain that recurs monthly. During pregnancy, endometriosis recedes, only to recur after the pregnancy when normal periods return.

During regular menstrual cycles, estrogen production rises around day 7 to 8 of the cycle and falls a day or so before your period begins. Progesterone production, on the other hand, starts after ovulation (two weeks before your period starts), reaching levels several hundred times greater than estrogen, and falls abruptly a day or so before the period. Using this concept as a model for women with endometriosis, transdermal progesterone can be given in doses similar to that of early pregnancy, starting at day 8 and continuing until day 26 of a usual 28-day cycle. Experience shows that this treatment is often effective in relieving the symptoms of endometriosis. Your goal is to find the lowest dose of progesterone necessary to control endometrial stimulation.

During the early weeks of pregnancy, progesterone production doubles or triples, from the normal 20 to 30 mg/day to 40 to 60 mg/day. These levels are easily reached using ¼ teaspoon of progesterone cream twice or three times a day during these 18 days of the cycle.

Improvement is usually noted after several months of progesterone cream used in this manner, but it can take up to six months for symptoms to be controlled, and even then they may not dissipate entirely. If the symptoms eventually disappear, the progesterone dose can be decreased gradually to find the lowest effective dose. (Otherwise use the dose that's most effective to control symptoms.) This must usually be continued until menopause is passed since recurrences are common if the progesterone protection is lowered too much. If a flare-up occurs, increase the dose to the previous effective level. High doses of progesterone cream make you sleepy; if this occurs, reduce the dose until the sleepiness goes away.

Uterine Fibroids

Women with fibroids are often estrogen dominant and have low progesterone levels. In women with smaller fibroids (the size of a tangerine or smaller), when progesterone is restored to normal levels, the fibroids often shrink a bit and stop growing, which is likely due to progesterone's ability to help speed up the clearance of estrogens from tissue. If this treatment can be continued through menopause, fibroid surgery can be avoided.

However, some fibroids, when they reach a certain "critical mass," are accompanied by degeneration or cell death in the interior part of the fibroid, and the ensuing inflammation results in the creation of more estrogens within the fibroid itself. It also contains growth factors that are stimulated by progesterone. Under these circumstances, surgical removal of the fibroid (myomectomy) or the uterus (hysterectomy) may become necessary. When you think of treating smaller fibroids you should be thinking in terms of keeping your estrogen levels as low as possible (without creating estrogen deficiency symptoms such as hot flashes and vaginal dryness), and when treating large fibroids, all hormones should be kept as low as possible.

The last thing you want to do if you have fibroids is to take estrogen, which will stimulate them to grow. If you're estrogen dominant then it's important to use a supplemental progesterone as recommended for a premeno-pausal woman. Sometimes this approach works to slow or stop fibroid growth, and sometimes it doesn't. It is worth a try. Reducing stress, increasing exercise, and reducing calories are also good strategies for slowing fibroid growth.

Fibroids almost always shrink and become inconsequential in menopausal women.

Breast Fibrocysts

Breast fibrocysts are fluid-filled fibrous cysts, usually tender and painful, more so during the last seven to eight days of the menstrual cycle, primarily due to estrogen dominance over a prolonged period of time. This is a sign that your ovaries are not producing enough progesterone. Breast fibrocysts respond remarkably well to transdermal progesterone, a fact which the French first recognized some 30 years ago.

Progesterone cream at 15 to 20 mg per day from ovulation until the day or two before your period starts will usually result in a return to normal breast tissue in three to four months. You can apply the progesterone cream to the breasts every few days if you find that helps. You can also take 400 IU of vitamin E at bedtime every night, as well as 300 mg of magnesium and 50 mg of vitamin B6 a day. For many women it helps to cut out caffeine (coffee and certain soft drinks) and reduce sugar and refined starches in the diet. Once the fibrocysts are under control, taper down the natural progesterone to the minimum dose needed to prevent recurrence.

Premenstrual Syndrome (PMS)

PMS usually involves a combination of hormone imbalance, stress, and higher levels of the hormone *cortisol*. Excessive cortisol not only reduces progesterone production but also competes with progesterone for common receptors, so you may need a higher progesterone dose than usual. For the first month or two, use as much as 50 mg of transdermal progesterone daily, starting mid-cycle (either day 12 or two weeks before your period is due).

You can also try gradually increasing the amount of cream you use, with small dabs at night starting on day 10 to 12 and gradually increasing to two dabs per day morning and night. Finish off the last three or four days with bigger dabs, or applying the cream three times a day. When symptoms subside, the dose may be reduced to find the lowest effective dose. Since PMS is a syndrome with multiple causative factors, it is wise to seek guidance in matters of stress management, diet, and other nutritional advice, such as is found in our book *What Your Doctor May* Not *Tell You About Premenopause.*

Premenstrual Migraine

Use natural progesterone during the 10 days before your period (day 16 to 26). If you feel the characteristic "aura" that usually precedes migraines, apply ¼ teaspoon of cream every three to four hours, until your symptoms cease (usually this happens in only one or two applications). You can also apply the cream directly to your neck or your temples.

In a Nutshell—Transdermal Hormones: When and How Much

(Note: These doses are for *transdermal* hormones, e.g., creams, gels, and oils.)

Getting each dab of cream to be exactly the right size isn't critical, because there's a buffering effect as the progesterone is absorbed into subcutaneous (under the skin) fat. The release of the hormone from body fat serves to make the progesterone effect relatively steady even if daily doses vary a little.

Progesterone

▶ Menopausal (not having menstrual cycles):10 to 20 mg of progesterone daily in divided doses (e.g., 5 to 10 mg twice daily) for 24 to 26 consecutive days a month, stopping for four to five days each month.

▶ Premenopausal (having menstrual cycles): 20 to 30 mg progesterone for the two weeks before menstruation begins.

Estrogen

▶ Menopausal: Patches are 0.25 to 0.05 mg; Bi-est cream is usually 0.1 to 0.2 mg of estradiol and 0.8 mg of estriol daily, and then adjust according to salivary hormone level tests and symptoms. As long as estrogen levels are kept low enough not to stimulate tissue buildup in the uterus, causing a period, it can be taken daily. Estrogen should never be taken without progesterone, even if you have no uterus.

▶ Premenopausal: If you're having periods, you're making enough estrogen. If you're having irregular periods, work with your doctor to decide whether estrogen is needed.

Testosterone

▶ Menopausal: Creams/gels, 0.1 to 1 mg daily or every other day.

▶ Premenopausal: Measure saliva hormone levels first and if testosterone levels are truly deficient, use smallest dose possible to alleviate symptoms.

Questions and Answers About Using Natural Progesterone Cream

Q: Will progesterone cream raise the levels of my other hormones?

A: This has been extensively tested by Dr. David Zava of ZRT Lab using saliva hormone level tests and the answer is no, progesterone cream does not raise the levels of other hormones. The body does use endogenous (made in the body) progesterone to create other hormones, but this does not occur with supplemental progesterone. However, the use of supplemental progesterone in someone who is deficient will keep estrogen receptors working efficiently, and it will improve thyroid function.

Q: If I'm menopausal and take progesterone, will my periods start again?

A: Not usually. The buildup of blood in the uterus is primarily a function of estrogen. At menopause, your production of estrogen does not fall to zero; it falls to a level just below that needed for monthly periods. It is likely, however, that your progesterone production is very close to zero. Without progesterone, estrogen receptors are less sensitive. When progesterone is resumed, estrogen receptors become more sensitive—that is, more likely to respond to estrogen. Thus some women may notice that after a week or two of progesterone some vaginal bleeding may occur due to their own estrogen. At that point, you can stop the progesterone for a week and then start up again for three weeks, as you would if you were still menstruating. The cycle should be three weeks on progesterone and one week off. During the week off progesterone, there may be some bleeding. This is due to the persistence of estrogen production, which will diminish over time. This is one of the reasons to stop progesterone for a few days each month: It allows the estrogen-induced blood buildup to be shed if it's there.

Later, when no monthly bleeding occurs, the progesterone can be continued on a calendar basis: 26 to 28 days of progesterone and then stopping for the remainder of the month. One easy way to remember this is to stop using the progesterone on the last day of every month, and start it on the fourth or fifth of the month. In cases of persistent spotting or vaginal bleeding (more than three months), consult your physician.

If you're taking estrogen, having a monthly period or spotting may be an indication that you're using too much estrogen. Try reducing the dose by half.

Q: Can I use natural progesterone if I'm taking birth control pills?

A: The honest answer to the above question is that we just don't know for sure. An educated guess is that the more potent progestins in the birth control pills will block progesterone from its receptors, but progesterone has many effects in different parts of the body, so it could have some benefit anyway. On the other hand, it isn't clear whether progesterone may interfere with the action of oral contraceptives. It is our hope that researchers can answer this question in the near future.

Q: What is the recommended dosage and timing of progesterone cream for women who are breast-feeding?

A: First, under the "if it ain't broke don't fix it" axiom, progesterone cream is not recommended postpartum unless it's needed. On the other hand, women suffering from the baby blues often benefit a great deal from a little progesterone. It's ideal if you can talk to your doctor about this, but generally, those who aren't having periods can use it three out of four weeks of the month, and those who are having periods can use it for the two weeks of the monthly cycle prior to menstruation. In both cases, a lower dose of 10 to 15 mg daily should suffice. It's ideal to use it in a divided dose, half in the morning and half before bed. Healthy young nursing mothers with good ovarian function shouldn't need to use it for very long once they begin menstruation again.

Also keep in mind that good nutrition and plenty of rest are essential to postpartum recovery.

Q: What if I have irregular bleeding?

A: Women who are perimenopausal are more than likely to have irregular periods, shorter or longer periods, heavier or lighter periods, and spotting in between periods. This is part of the menopausal transition for many women and you just have to go with the flow (so to speak).

If you start using progesterone cream and find that you're suddenly experiencing spotting between periods, there could be a number of reasons. The most common reason is too high a dose of progesterone. The second most common reason is that your timing is off. If you've had a 24-day cycle for years and suddenly start using progesterone as if you're on a 28-day cycle, your body can become confused. That's why I now recommend that women who are having periods figure out when to start the progesterone cream each month by calculating when their next period is due and counting back two weeks.

Q: My symptoms return when I stop using the progesterone each month. Do I *have* to take the break?

A: It's ideal to stop for four to six days, but some women stop for only three to four days and that seems to work. There are two very good reasons for stopping. One is that your progesterone receptors need to be refreshed occasionally. If they're getting a nonstop progesterone message they will conclude that there's too much progesterone in the system and start to shut down. If your receptors start to shut down, the progesterone you're taking won't be used and your symptoms will start to return. This is the same thing that happens when you use too much progesterone.

The other reason to stop for a week is to make sure there's no buildup of tissue in the uterus that needs to be shed—in other words, if your body needs to have a period, this gives it the opportunity. Allowing tissue to build up in the uterus long term without a period could put you at risk for uterine cancer. This is why it's particularly important to take the days off if you're also using estrogen.

Where to Find Natural Progesterone

At this time, natural progesterone cream is available over the counter and by prescription at compounding pharmacies. You can usually find it in health food stores, and it's easy to find on the Internet. Be sure that you're getting the real thing. If the label says "wild yam extract," don't buy the product without calling or e-mailing the company and confirming that it contains the necessary amount of progesterone and not diosgenin or dioscorea, which are precursors of progesterone in the laboratory but do *not* convert to progesterone in the body.

Your doctor can order a progesterone cream from a compounding pharmacist, but be careful of the 10 percent creams that contain very high amounts of progesterone. Taking a higher-than-recommended dose does not contribute to hormone balance. The optimal amount is a 1.6 to 2 percent progesterone cream by weight, with about 450 to 500 mg of progesterone per ounce. In $1/4$ teaspoon of cream this amounts to about 15 to 20 mg of progesterone.

Many natural progesterone creams contain ingredients other than progesterone that may be active, including "wild yam extract," which is usually diosgenin, as well as a variety of herbs and aromatic oils. We do not know which are active and which aren't, or what biochemical effects these ingredients may or may not have, nor do we know what effect they may have when used by women who are pregnant or nursing. In an extensive screening of hundreds of herbs traditionally used for hormonal imbalances, Dr. David Zava has yet to identify one that has activity similar to natural progesterone. For this reason, we feel that progesterone creams containing herbs should be avoided by women who are trying to get pregnant, who are pregnant, or who are nursing. These women are advised to use one of the creams that contain only progesterone as the active ingredient. (This is not to say that the other ingredients aren't helpful for women with hormone imbalances—we suspect they probably *are*.)

Some herbs have traditionally been used to stop pregnancy (abortifacients), induce menstrual periods (emmenagogue), or to induce labor. In his research, Dr. Zava has found that these herbs interact with progesterone receptors but do not activate the receptor in the same manner as natural progesterone. In fact, many behave more like an anti-progesterone, which is consistent with the traditional uses mentioned above.

A progesterone cream that feels grainy or sandy probably means the progesterone has precipitated out. We recommend that you return or exchange it. We do not recommend creams that contain other hormones besides progesterone.

The Resources section at the back of this book lists progesterone creams that contain our recommended dose of progesterone. Most of those listed are companies we've known for years, and we offer the list as a service to our readers with no charge to or compensation from the companies. There are plenty of perfectly good progesterone creams that aren't on this list, many of them private label versions of these creams. Due to space limitations we can't list them all. Neither of the authors of this book sell (or sold) progesterone cream or make any money from the sale of any progesterone cream.

Other Causes of Hormone Imbalance

Hormones and their glands do not operate in a vacuum; they have complex and important interactions with every other system in your body. We're all familiar by now with the basics of good health: eat wholesome food, get plenty of exercise and sleep, and manage stress. We could often get away with an unhealthy lifestyle in our twenties, and maybe even our early thirties, but by our mid-thirties we start to pay the price, and by our fifties it will cause illness. We have covered the topics of diet, exercise, sleep, and adrenal fatigue in great detail in our other books, but in this chapter we want to address some of the not-so-obvious causes of poor health and hormone imbalances. These causes fall under general categories of diet, stress, toxins, and lifestyle, but we want to give you a fresh new perspective based on the latest research that will help you improve your own health. Let's begin with an example of someone who thought they were doing everything right for their health.

The Queen of Denial

A friend once phoned me, and she lamented over the fact that she couldn't seem to lose weight. She worked out four days a week, two of them with a personal trainer. She didn't eat breakfast, ate a salad for lunch, and had meat and vegetables for dinner. "And still," she said, "I'm not dropping any weight and I'm tired all the time."

"What are you eating in the way of sugar?" I asked.

"Well, I probably drink three Cokes over the course of a day . . ."

As educated as my friend was about diet and exercise, it simply didn't compute for her that drinking three Cokes a day could keep the weight on and cause fatigue. It doesn't have any fat or carbohydrates, right? And all that caffeine should be giving her energy, right? No such luck.

Three Coca-Colas contain the equivalent of 18 teaspoons of sugar, and that can pack on the pounds and increase fatigue, even with all that caffeine. Carbohydrates are broken down into sugar in the body, so for those of you on a low-carb diet, sugar has the same effect as eating carbohydrates. (High-protein diets could also be called low-carbohydrate *and* low-sugar diets.) How about Diet Coke without the sugar? There's not one single study showing that diet sodas contribute to weight loss, and believe me, millions of dollars have been spent trying to prove this.

Then there was the letter I received from a woman who is a vegetarian, a supposedly healthy style of eating, and yet she is dealing with excess weight, fatigue, and chronic indigestion. She typically has a bagel with margarine or a sugar-free jam for breakfast; a banana midmorning; a salad with rice, beans, bread or chips for lunch; a protein bar or trail mix for an afternoon snack; and for dinner typically eats vegetables with beans, rice or some other grain, occasionally adding tofu or tempeh.

And of course there's the typical dietary scenario of the American Heart Association that includes low-fat proteins, simple carbohydrates, vegetables and sweets, but as Americans have followed these dictates they have become increasingly obese.

On the other side of the coin, I have a relative who cut sugar, refined carbohydrates, and alcohol almost entirely from her diet, but now allows herself plenty of butter; olive oil; a variety of quality protein such as meat, fish, chicken, and eggs; and a wide variety of vegetables and complex carbohydrates. No, she's not doing the extreme Atkins diet that heaps on the fat and shuns carbohydrates almost entirely. This is a much more balanced approach. She loves the new diet, and after decades of struggling with weight gain, she's been steadily dropping five to seven pounds a month for the past six months. She says that her "pep" is back and so is her sense of humor.

Food, Fat, Fatigue, and Insulin

Fat makes you fat, right? And calories are calories, regardless of where they come from. If only it were that simple. In truth, your body does very different things with fats, sugars, other carbohydrates, and proteins. It also responds differently depending on how you combine food groups. For example, a combination of fat, carbohydrate, and sugar (think pastries and cookies) can create blood sugar havoc, while fat, complex carbohydrates, and protein (think meat and whole grain rice) can create blood sugar stability. Stable blood sugar is one of the foundations of maintaining a healthy weight.

However, everything I'm about to say comes with one big caveat: moderation. *If you eat enormous amounts of food you're going to become enormous regardless of what diet you're on.* If you eat mostly white, doughy foods, your body is going to be white and doughy. None of the women I described above were overeating; they were eating in a way that encouraged their bodies to put on weight instead of losing or maintaining it.

Back to Food Basics

As most of you know, three basic kinds of foods are converted into fuel: proteins, fats, and carbohydrates. Proteins such as dairy products, meats, fish, and eggs are broken down into amino acids. Fats such as butter, cream, bacon, and oils are broken down into fatty acids. Carbohydrates—whether from cakes, candy, fruits, potatoes, grains, or starchy vegetables—are broken down into simple sugars. Misuse and abuse of sugars is where most Americans get their fat and their fatigue.

What Sugar Does in Your Body

Sugar enters the bloodstream in a form called glucose, the main source of fuel for the body, and especially the brain. The cells that ultimately use the glucose for fuel do not care whether it originally came from Ben and Jerry's ice cream or the carbohydrates in broccoli. What does dramatically affect your body is how fast the glucose enters the bloodstream. Ben and Jerry's will cause a quick, large surge in glucose, whereas broccoli will cause only the slightest rise over time. Excess glucose is toxic to the kidneys and other organs, and this is where insulin comes in. In response to rising glucose, the pancreas secretes the hormone insulin into the bloodstream. Insulin's job is to transport glucose out of the bloodstream and into your cells, which is why a big surge of glucose causes a big release of insulin. However, too much insulin is also toxic, so your body works hard to maintain balance. Researchers estimate that there are as many as 20,000 insulin receptors or more per cell.

As your glucose level gradually falls after a meal or snack, the amount of insulin in the blood also falls. At any given time the blood can carry about an hour's supply of glucose. Any glucose that is not needed for immediate energy is converted into glycogen and stored in the liver and muscles. When it is required for energy, the liver turns the glycogen back into glucose. The body can store only enough glycogen to last for several hours of moderate activity. Finally, when its glycogen is used up, the body turns to stored fat for fuel. When glucose levels rise, your body stops using stored fat. Thus, you can understand why my friend who drinks Cokes all day long isn't losing weight—her body has no need to burn its fat because she's constantly feeding it instant glucose!

Insulin Resistance

Inside the insulin receptor is an enzyme called tyrosine kinase (TK). Once activated by insulin this enzyme triggers a cascade of events that open channels through which glucose can enter the cells to be stored or used for energy. When cells become insulin resistant, the channels do not open and the glucose fails to gain entry into the cells. Insulin resistance causes glucose to build up in the bloodstream, which in turn signals the pancreas to make more insulin. The end result is higher-than-normal levels of both insulin and glucose in the bloodstream, which promotes the formation of fat and causes abnormal cholesterol, high triglycerides, high blood pressure, and eventually, clogged arteries. In fact, when you're insulin resistant, the only cells in the body that benefit from excess sugar are cancer cells, which happily use it for energy and growth.

Researchers in the prestigious Framingham Study estimate that as much as 60 percent of heart disease in women is caused by insulin resistance. The constellation of symptoms caused by insulin resistance has come to be known as Syndrome X, a term coined by Gerald Reaven, M.D., a Stanford University researcher.

Over time, insulin resistance causes muscle cells to weaken due to lack of fuel, and thus begins a vicious cycle of less exercise, more weight gain, and more insulin resistance.

As fat increases and muscle decreases, the body loses more and more of its ability to burn fuel efficiently and metabolism slows to a crawl.

Insulin resistance is often the precursor to type 2 diabetes. Clearly, eating sugars and simple carbohydrates when you're insulin resistant will only make it worse.

We don't know the exact mechanisms that cause insulin resistance, but we do know that insulin resistance, abdominal obesity, and stress tend to go hand-in-hand. The high cortisol levels caused by stress tend to cause abdominal obesity, which in turn is one of the hallmarks of insulin resistance. So if you tend to head for the ice cream, pastries, and cookies when you're stressed, it may be time to look for a different coping mechanism.

And by the way, you can be slim and still be insulin resistant, with all of the fatigue and other damage still occurring in the body. My guess is that chronic stress combined with genetic predisposition and a sugar-laden diet are the common threads of insulin resistance.

Slowing the Glucose Train

Clearly, big surges of glucose are the foundation of fat and fatigue. So how do we slow the glucose train? The most obvious answer is to not eat sugar and refined carbohydrates. But getting enough protein and eating some fat can also help, and that's why diets that shun protein or fat can cause weight gain and fatigue.

Whole grains, fiber, protein, and fat can all help slow things down. Complex carbohydrates such as those found in whole grains, fresh vegetables, nuts, seeds, and beans tend to break down slowly in the gut and cause a very gradual rise in blood sugar. Complex carbohydrates tend to be higher in fiber, which also slows down the digestive process.

The body breaks proteins down into amino acids, some of which are stored in the liver for the manufacture of glucagon, which allows the release of glycogen, which you'll remember is the body's backup system when glucose levels start to fall after a meal. No protein means no glycogen, which means no backup glucose, which means intense sugar/carbohydrate cravings as the body signals for more glucose—fast!

This is why the vegetarian who eats a bagel for breakfast (a simple carbohydrate that breaks down quickly into glucose); a banana (fruit sugar); a salad with bread (more simple carbohydrates); a protein bar (they're all loaded with sugar); or trail mix (raisins are very sweet); and more carbohydrates with dinner, but very little protein throughout the day, is gaining weight and feeling tired. She'd be better off having a piece of whole grain toast with butter and an egg for breakfast; tofu with her salad for lunch, and fish for dinner, for example.

When I talk about fats as good foods, I'm not talking

about the trans-fatty acids (hydrogenated oils) found in many processed foods—please avoid those. Any food made with hydrogenated or partially hydrogenated oils will say so on the label. These fats are rarely made by Mother Nature, so if you're eating whole, unprocessed foods, you need not worry about avoiding them.

Fat slows the glucose train for a number of reasons. As fat hits the taste buds, it sends signals to the rest of the gastrointestinal system that rich fuel and calories are coming, and that creates "I'm satisfied" or satiety signals. Fats—and especially saturated fats—are easy to digest, are burned for fuel quickly and efficiently, and tend to speed up metabolism in general while slowing the digestion of sugars.

As long as you consume fat in moderation, your body is very good at ridding itself of excess fats, including cholesterol.

Find What Works Best for *You*

Always keep in mind that we're each unique in our genetic makeup and biochemistry, and what works well for one person may not work for another. One person may thrive on meat and vegetables, while another may thrive on fish and rice, and yet another may need a minimum of protein and more carbohydrates. If you keep the above principles in mind, you can eat in a way that's very satisfying and yet doesn't keep increasing your weight.

Pick and Choose Your Salmon

On the surface, salmon appears to be one of the ultimate health foods: it's a great source of high-quality protein and the important omega-3 fats, and it's not overly expensive. However, the popularity of salmon has spurred the development of farmed salmon raised in crowded conditions. Intensive farming techniques tend to be good for profits but not so good for the consumer. Cows, pigs, and chickens kept in densely packed feedlots and cages must be fed antibiotics to keep disease from taking over, and now farmed Atlantic salmon has joined that group.

Virtually all of the Atlantic salmon that you buy in the supermarket comes from farms where the salmon are raised in crowded floating cages. To keep disease and parasite levels down, pesticides, antibiotics, and other drugs are dumped directly into the ocean. Salmon farms also produce a huge volume of feces that pollute the ocean for miles around and sea lice that infect the already-threatened population of wild Atlantic salmon.

According to the World Health Organization, salmon farms use more antibiotics by weight than any other farmed animal. Furthermore, their fat is lower in the beneficial essential fatty acids than wild salmon.

What you can do as a consumer is avoid Atlantic salmon altogether, and look for wild Pacific salmon, which is fresh from April through October and available frozen year-round.

Dietary Balance Guidelines in a Nutshell

▶ Minimize sugar and refined carbohydrates (e.g., sodas, cookies, chips, ice cream, white bread, white rice, pasta).

▶ Have some protein with every meal or snack (e.g., meat, fish, eggs, cheese, nuts and seeds, tofu).

▶ Eat plenty of high-fiber foods (e.g., vegetables, fruits, whole grain breads, brown rice).

▶ Avoid trans-fatty acids (e.g., hydrogenated oils).

▶ Eat fats in moderation but don't avoid them— they help slow digestion and send "I'm full" signals to the brain.

Insulin and Hormones

What does all this have to do with hormones? Chronically high insulin stimulates the ovaries to produce more androgens (male hormones), which is a primary cause of polycystic ovary syndrome (PCOS). Symptoms of PCOS can include extreme pain and discomfort in the middle of a menstrual cycle (around ovulation), excessive hair on the face, legs, and arms, and hair loss on the head. Not surprisingly, we have an epidemic of PCOS among girls in their teens and women in their twenties, owing to the typical American diet high in sugars and refined carbohydrates.

Women with PCOS generally don't ovulate, and thus they don't produce progesterone, which can potentially lead to estrogen dominance and perhaps breast cancer.

In a Nutshell—How Overeating Junk Food Early in Life May Increase Breast Cancer Risk

Overeating junk food makes you fat. Increased body fat and lack of exercise lead to insulin resistance. (Smoking makes it happen faster.) Insulin resistance leads to further craving of sugary carbohydrates to generate energy for the body. More insulin is released in response to increased carbohydrate intake, leading to more weight gain. More fat leads to more estrogens, which, in turn, leads to earlier breast development and onset of menstruation. Earlier onset of menstruation leads to more ovulatory cycles and a greater lifetime exposure to estrogens without adequate progesterone. A greater lifetime exposure to estrogens without the protection of progesterone increases breast cancer risk.

Simultaneously, increased consumption of simple carbohydrates, coupled with insulin resistance, leads to polycystic ovaries and lack of ovulation during menstrual cycles, resulting in excess production of androgens and estrogens, and inadequate production of progesterone. Excessive estrogen production in the absence of progesterone production leads to estrogen dominance and increased breast cancer risk.

Use of contraceptive hormones (often used by M.D.s to treat PCOS) increases insulin resistance, exacerbating many of the problems above.

Insulin Resistance Combined with Menopause

Symptoms of PCOS, high androgens, and insulin resistance can also be symptoms of approaching menopause. Higher androgens and an increased waist-to-hip ratio (fat around the middle) are significant risk factors for breast cancer because the increased fat around the waist results in a greater capacity to form estrogens from androgens, further increasing breast cancer risk. In fact, it may not be the increase in androgens per se that increases breast cancer risk, but rather the enhanced capacity, caused by insulin resistance, to convert them to estrogens in fat tissue adjacent to the breast cells. At the same time, the drop in the cyclic production of estrogen and progesterone, as well as in androgens such as DHEA, can also increase the chances of developing insulin resistance, and the lowered progesterone contributes to estrogen dominance.

Prescription Drugs That Can Cause High Blood Sugar

Here are some prescription drugs that can cause hyperglycemia, or high blood sugar.

Calcium channel blockers for heart arrhythmias [nifedipine (Procardia), nicardipine (Cardene), diltiazem (Cardizem), verapamil]

Antihypertensives that lower blood pressure (clonidine, diazoxide, diuretics)

Corticosteroids (Prednisone)

Epinephrine (bronchodilators, decongestants)
Heparin to prevent blood clotting
Thyroid drugs for low thyroid (Levoxine, Synthroid)
Morphine
Nicotine
Pentamidine for the treatment of pneumonia
Phenytoin for the treatment of seizures (Dilantin)
Antituberculosis drugs (rifampin [Rifadin, Rimac-
    tane], isoniazid [Laniazid, Nydrazid])

Stress, Fatigue, and Cortisol

We received a letter from a woman named Anne that il-
lustrates the many ways that stress can affect our hormone levels and our health:

> About 10 years ago I was leaving my marriage, moving
> out on my own, and building a new career. I was in my
> early forties, had very little money and few friends, and
> my family lived on the other side of the country.
> Shortly after moving out I started to experience a lot of
> fatigue and mental fogginess—not what I needed to
> start life over! The more tired and foggy I got, the
> harder I tried to be "good." I tried to force myself to
> work harder and to exercise; I restricted my diet to veg-

etables, whole grains, and soy, and eventually became so ill that I could barely move. My blood pressure was very low and my muscles were so weak I could barely stand up straight. I went to doctors who patted me on the head and offered me antidepressants like Prozac and anti-anxiety drugs like Ativan, but I knew that wasn't the answer. I found myself going out to a coffee shop around midmorning and loading up on cinnamon buns and coffee to try to get through part of a day. Finally a friend insisted that I go listen to a speaker who talked about progesterone, and afterwards I told him my story. He exclaimed, "You need to use progesterone and eat more meat and salt! And stop exercising so much!" I did, and my health improved dramatically, but I still had a sense of underlying fatigue and fogginess that I fought with coffee.

A few years later I got a bad case of poison oak that wouldn't go away, and an alternatively minded doctor put me on 20 mg of hydrocortisone a day for a week. What a change! Suddenly my energy was up and my head was clear. I felt like my old self. My doctor explained that this was an indication that I had adrenal fatigue and put me on a regimen of vitamins and herbs to build up my adrenals, along with 5 mg of hydrocortisone twice a day. This worked really well, but I used the extra energy to take on more work than I was capable of reasonably handling and got involved in an intense relationship that had a lot of ups and downs. I stayed up late working and had trouble getting out of bed in the morning, and eventually I started to go downhill again.

Next my doctor put me on thyroid medication, which again helped, and again I took advantage of the newly found energy to overdo it. When that stopped being effective, I turned to testosterone, and it helped for a while, but that wore off too. I'm also eating a diet of mostly vegetables, meat, and fish, and that's helped a lot, but it wasn't the whole answer.

Dr. Lee, I've finally realized that the common denominator over the years has been my insistence on overdoing it and stressing myself out. Whenever my energy increases, I use it to push myself harder. I rarely rest except when forced to by exhaustion. I rarely take vacations and every time I do I get sick afterwards. I push and push and push myself to do more, when what I need to do is chill (as my young friends would say)!

Recently I've started getting into bed by 10 p.m. and taking weekends off. I also take numerous little breaks during the day to take a few deep breaths, step back from my day-to-day life, and get a larger perspective. It's made a huge difference—as much as any of the hormones and vitamins have. Not that I'm going to give up my progesterone, but I've realized that boosting my hormones and nutrients isn't going to help unless I also discipline myself to relax. Sounds like a contradiction, but it's true!

My guess is that many of you can relate to Anne's story. Baby boomers tend to be a generation driven to relentlessly strive to have it all, but that comes at a cost. Let's look more closely at what happens when we constantly flog our adrenal glands in the process of pursuing perfection.

The Adrenal Hormones

The adrenal glands respond to any stressors that increase energy requirements. Fasting, infection, intense exercise, pain, or emotional or mental stress stimulate the secretion of a releasing hormone from the hypothalamus in the brain, which tells the adrenals to secrete extra cortisol and other stress hormones. There's also a regular daily cycle of cortisol release into the bloodstream, with peaks in the morning and late afternoon and lows in mid-afternoon and during deep sleep.

Cortisol is needed for nearly all dynamic processes in the body, from blood pressure regulation and kidney function, to glucose levels and fat building, muscle building, protein synthesis, thyroid function, and immune function.

Cortisol is extremely important to survival when stress of any sort is present. If our lives were stress-free, a lack of cortisol would not be life-threatening. But without the corticosteroids, we can't survive even the slightest stress. People who have had their adrenal glands removed or whose adrenals don't make enough cortisol are in danger of death from even mild illness. These people must use cortisol replacement for the rest of their lives, increasing their dose at any sign of extra stress or infection. Many of you are in a less extreme version of this scenario, with tired adrenals that have trouble responding appropriately to stress.

Excessive cortisol, on the other hand, creates a broad range of undesirable side effects including weight gain around the waist; elevated blood glucose, which leads to insulin resistance; high blood pressure; osteoporosis; easy bruising; a susceptibility to fungal infections; and disorders of the immune system.

Chronic stress leads to chronic high levels of cortisol in the bloodstream, which creates a need for more hormones (e.g., thyroid, insulin, progesterone, testosterone) in order to do the same job. According to Dr. David Zava, who has studied the interaction of cortisol and hormones:

> When cortisol is high the brain is less sensitive to estrogens. That's why you can have a postmenopausal woman with reasonable amounts of estrogen, but when you put her under a stressor and her cortisol rises, she'll get hot flashes, which are a symptom of estrogen deficiency. She really doesn't have an estrogen deficiency, the brain sensors have just been altered. If you then drive the estrogen levels up with supplementation to treat the hot flashes, she'll start getting symptoms of estrogen dominance like weight gain in the hips, water retention, and

moodiness. And the hot flashes usually don't go away. This is why you often can't effectively treat someone with hormonal imbalance symptoms such as hot flashes by simply adding what seems to be the missing hormone, be it thyroid, progesterone, estrogen, or testosterone. If your cortisol is chronically high you'll have overall resistance to your hormones. It's essential to address the stress factor if you want to achieve hormone balance.

Chronic cortisol exposure in high concentrations is toxic to brain cells and can cause short-term memory loss. A lifetime of high cortisol levels may be a primary contributor to Alzheimer's disease and senile dementia. High cortisol is also a primary cause of osteoporosis because it blocks the bone-building effects of progesterone.

Like the other hormones, cortisol is essential to good health and even to life, but in excess or deficiency can be harmful. Maintaining healthy cortisol levels isn't just a matter of tweaking your biochemistry with this or that diet, hormone, vitamin or mineral (although that can be a big help!). Balanced cortisol is also a matter of respecting yourself and caring enough about your health to get plenty of sleep, some moderate exercise and fresh air, and to bring some relaxation, laughter, and fun into your life.

You can easily test your cortisol levels with a saliva test. A normal morning saliva hormone level for cortisol for a perimenopausal woman is 3 to 8 ng/ml, and by 10 at night it's 0.5 to 1.5 ng/ml. Very early in the morning when you're in a deep sleep it goes even lower, so if you're not sleeping properly and resting, your cortisol rhythms will be thrown out of balance.

Take Your Vitamin ZZZ's

It may seem self-evident that getting enough sleep is important to your health, but University of Chicago researchers have honed in on some interesting specifics. In comparing a group of men and women who habitually slept 6.5 hours a night with a comparable group who slept about 8 hours, they found that the short sleepers had 50 percent more insulin resistance than the others. Insulin resistance predisposes you to diabetes, heart disease, and hormonal imbalance.

In another experiment, sleep-deprived men had greatly reduced levels of leptin, a hormone that tells the brain when you're full and regulates energy balance. Low leptin levels can cause overeating and a slow metabolism that will predispose to obesity.

Other research has shown an increase in substances that increase inflammation (a key factor in heart disease) in sleep-deprived volunteers, and rats deprived of sleep show elevated levels of stress hormones.

Before you get stressed out about not getting enough sleep, remember that there are no hard and fast rules about how much sleep you need as an individual. Some people thrive on seven hours a night, while others need eight or nine.

Some of our greatest thinkers, such as Albert Einstein, got minimal sleep at night but took naps in the afternoon. Find out what works for you, but do take your vitamin zzz's!

Toxic Exposure

As we explained in the chapter on estrogen, xenoestrogens are not-found-in-nature estrogens with toxic estrogen effects on the human body. Xenoestrogens are found in most pesticides, plastics, acetones (e.g., fingernail polish remover), and in industrial pollutants such as PCBs. They tend to be very potent and toxic and aren't easily eliminated from the body. Once again, you can get details on how xenoestrogens affect you in our other books, but here's a short list of how to avoid them in your own home.

Clean Up Your House to Clean Up Your Hormones

• Throw away all pesticides, herbicides, fungicides. Take a class in organic gardening and read up on natural pest control. *Do not* tent your house and fumigate it with pesticides, or "bomb" it, or have your lawn sprayed with chemicals.

• Throw away nail polish and nail polish remover; it's toxic both when you breathe it and when you put it on your nails. There is no safe nail polish at this time. It is particularly damaging to allow young girls to use nail polish.

• Don't use fabric softeners; this puts petrochemicals directly into the air and onto your skin, which is quite capable of absorbing all kinds of substances.

• Most scented products and perfumes are petrochemically based, and when you inhale them they go directly to your brain. Don't use petrochemically based perfumes or air fresheners. Try some of the natural aromatic oils and combinations if you want to change how you, your house, or your car smell. In the same vein, use unscented laundry soaps and naturally scented shampoos and conditioners.

• A new home can be a toxic soup of noxious gases coming from glues, fiberboard, new carpet, and new paint. If your new home makes you feel sick it is *not* all in your head; have the air tested. Chances are it's loaded with formaldehyde and solvent fumes. When you're pregnant or have an infant, it's not a good idea to move into a newly built home, remodel, or even paint. This can be challenging for a pregnant woman when the nesting instinct kicks in, but first consider the future health of your baby.

Are You Allergic to Fake Fragrances? Just Because It Smells Good Doesn't Mean It's Good for You

Jennifer was shopping in the mall and stepped into an elevator with another woman who was wearing a generous amount of perfume. By the time she got off the elevator, Jennifer was feeling, as she described it, "stuffy, dizzy, and disconnected." She tried to continue shopping, but wound up going home and sleeping it off. Jennifer has since discovered that she's allergic to petrochemically based fragrances. She tries to avoid elevators as well as scented cosmetics, laundry detergents, fabric softeners, air fresheners, and scented candles.

Next time you're about to apply a few drops of perfume to your wrists, consider whether it might adversely affect your health, or the health of someone else. That fatigue or brain fog you're experiencing may be due to a hormonal imbalance or not getting enough sleep the night before, or it could be due to an allergy to commercial fragrances. You may think that your expensive perfume is made from a lovely field of flowers or an exotic potion of herbs, but chances are good it's derived primarily from petroleum. The majority of perfumes, hair care products, and other cosmetic lotions and potions are made with petrochemicals that can have effects ranging from skin irritation to outright toxicity.

While the FDA requires that the labels on personal-care products list the ingredients, "fragrance" is a catch-all word for a veritable stew of chemicals that are unregulated and largely untested. The most common reaction to these chemicals is dermatitis (skin rash), which can include itching, swelling, redness, and even blisters.

Synthetic fragrances can also cause or aggravate asthma and allergies, particularly in children. How many children are suffering from asthma because their clothes are washed with heavily scented fabric softeners or because their bedroom contains a plug-in air freshener?

Phthalates, which are well known to be carcinogenic, are common ingredients in "fragrances." Dibutyl phthalate (DBP) is a reproductive toxin, which means it could be harmful to a developing fetus.

Meaningless Labels

If you visit your health food store, personal-care products labeled "organic," "natural," or "hypoallergenic" must be safe, right? Unfortunately not. While foods have strict guidelines regarding the use of the terms, personal-care products do not, making these labels virtually meaningless. A product with one organic ingredient out of twenty can label itself "organic."

Naturally Scented

If you enjoy perfumes, try those made with essential oils. To be sure that's what you're getting, you'll need to find products that list each ingredient. You can even use a tiny drop of a pure essential oil, although some of those can be irritating to the skin, particularly citrus, mint, and eucalyptus.

If You're Allergic

If you're highly sensitive to synthetic fragrances, it can become difficult to even venture out of the house. Fake smells are everywhere: the supermarket aisles that sell cleaning products and air fresheners, gift shops with scented products of every description, beauty salons with hair sprays and gels, cosmetics counters in department stores, cleaning products used in restaurants and office buildings—even at the car wash they'll spritz the inside of your car with offensive air freshener.

Does this mean you need to be a housebound victim to this cultural obsession with how things smell? For most people, the answer is no. Although you would be smart to avoid having synthetic fragrances in your home or work environment, most of us can tolerate occasional exposure to them. Sensitivities and allergies are generally caused by an overreactive immune system that perceives these petrochemicals as harmful invaders. (Okay, they are, but most immune systems will ignore them unless constantly exposed.)

The best way to calm an overreactive immune system is to support your adrenal glands. The foundation of healthy adrenals is stress management, enough sleep, and hormone balance. Vitamin C, licorice root, and pantothenic acid (a form of vitamin B5) can all support the adrenals, and there are many vitamin formulas made specifically for that purpose.

Exercise Is a Foundation of Hormone Balance

Last but not least, exercise is an essential component of maintaining hormone balance. In fact, if you've been leading a couch potato existence and ignored all of the other recommendations in this book but did embark on a regular exercise program, your hormone balance would improve dramatically within a matter of months.

Most of our chronic illnesses, such as heart disease, arthritis, and cancer, can be traced to lack of exercise, and the obesity caused by lack of exercise. The human body is built for movement. Every system in your body, from your organs, circulatory and lymph systems, to your muscles and bones, performs best for you when it is moved and stretched regularly.

You don't need to take up jogging or go to the gym to get adequate exercise. For most people, a brisk 20- to 30-minute walk every day or so will do the job. Gardening, raking leaves, mowing the lawn, and shoveling snow are all good exercise. Or try swimming, bike riding, tennis, or golf (without the cart). Yoga and the Chinese movement exercises such as tai chi and qi gong are excellent for keeping the body toned and supple. Some people dance, some take aerobics classes, some use exercise videos, others have exercise machines. What's important is to find a form (or forms) of exercise that you enjoy, and then make it a near daily habit. (For most people, planning daily exercise results in actually getting it three to four days a week!)

Other Benefits of Exercise

- *Stronger bones:* A regular program of weight-bearing exercise will help strengthen bones. Walking, running, jogging, and weight lifting will build bone, increase muscle mass, and create better balance and coordination.

- *A better cholesterol profile:* Aerobic exercise, which is the kind that gets your heart pumping, can lower your "bad" LDL cholesterol and raise your "good" HDL cholesterol.

- *Lower blood pressure:* People who exercise are 34 percent less likely to develop high blood pressure. A brisk half-hour walk three or four times a week can lower blood pressure by 3 to 15 points in three months.

- *Improves circulation:* Movement helps move blood through the body and helps move toxins out of the body through sweating and lymph drainage. Improved blood circulation can help with heart disease, diabetes, and arthritis.

- *Prevent and alleviate depression:* Exercise can increase levels of brain chemicals called endorphins, which create a sense of well-being and relieve pain, which can help keep depression at bay.

- *Healthier joints:* Exercise keeps your joints flexible, increases muscle strength around joints to give them greater support, and helps move the toxic by-products of inflammation out of the joints by improving your circulation.

- *Supports the immune system:* Exercise in moderation supports the immune system by increasing white blood cells, which help the body fight infection.

Conclusion

At the beginning of this book, we gave you Dr. Lee's Three Rules for Hormone Replacement Therapy:

Rule 1: Use Hormones Only if You Need Them (e.g., if they are measurably low and/or you have clear symptoms)

Rule 2: Use Bioidentical Hormones Rather Than Synthetic Hormones

Rule 3: Use Hormones Only in Dosages That Create Hormone Balance

Whether you're just starting to use natural hormones, or you've been using them for a while and feel you need to make some changes to get back on track, start by referring back to these rules, and then refer to the chapters in the book that apply, or skim through some of the lists for guidance.

You don't have to wait until you have a healthy lifestyle to start using natural hormones. Correcting a hormonal imbalance can help you feel better, so that it's easier to put energy and attention into positive change in other areas of your life. Likewise, each small step that you take to improve your eating habits, your sleep, and so on, will make it easier to achieve hormone balance.

As you strive for hormone balance, remember that it is woven into the overall fabric of a healthy lifestyle that includes wholesome food, moderate exercise, enough sleep, avoidance of toxins, and stress management. These practical and seemingly simple threads of our day-to-day lives are truly the foundation of good health and hormone balance.

Protect Your Right to Use Natural Hormones

This book is being published at a time when many of the drug companies that make synthetic hormones are attempting to preserve their market share by criticizing natural hormones and hoping to make them go away. The good news is that most people aren't listening. Thousands of doctors are confidently and competently prescribing bioidentical hormones, and millions of women are happily and healthily using them. If you're one of those happy, healthy women, this would be a good time to e-mail your representatives in Washington, D.C., and voice your support for natural hormones! To e-mail your United States congressman go to http://www.house.gov/writerep/. To e-mail your United States senator go to http://www.senate.gov/.

Resources

General Information
www.johnleemd.com and **www.hopkinstestkits.com.**
These are the websites of Pat Lee and Virginia Hopkins, respectively. On them, you'll find a wealth of information related to natural hormone balance.

www.hopkinshealthwatch.com. This is where you can read and sign up for the "Hopkins Health Watch," a free e-mail newsletter by Virginia Hopkins about the latest in natural hormone and nutrition news, including interviews with experts in the field, updates on research, warnings about dangerous prescription drugs and their interactions, and much more!

Saliva Hormone Testing
ZRT Laboratory, 1815 NW 169th Place, Suite 5050, Beaverton, OR 97006, (503) 466-2445, www.salivatest .com. This is Dr. David Zava's company, a pioneer in saliva hormone testing. You can also order ZRT saliva test kits from www.johnleemd.com and www.hopkinstestkits.com.

Progesterone Creams

This is a free list that is updated regularly on www .johnleemd.com and www.hopkinstestkits.com. It is based on our knowledge of the companies and their products, but we cannot guarantee that any of these creams contain Dr. Lee's recommended doses. There are many good creams available that are not on this list.

Dr. Lee never endorsed or recommended any one progesterone cream nor did he make money from the sale of any progesterone cream. Companies that state or imply otherwise on their websites or elsewhere should be avoided.

Alternative Medicine Network, 601 16th Street, #C-#105, Golden, CO 80401, toll-free (877) 753-5424, e-mail: sales @altmednetwork.net, www.altmednetwork.net. They make Awakening Woman Natural Progesterone Cream, which contains only progesterone as its active ingredient.

Bio-Nutritional Formulas, 106 E. Jericho Turnpike, P.O. Box 311, Mineola, NY 11501, (800) 950-8484. Pure-Gest cream.

Broadmoore Labs, Inc., 3875 Telegraph Road/294, Ventura, CA 93003, (800) 822-3712. Makers of Natra-Gest (regular and fragrance-free), no parabens. Consultations available.

Dr. Helen Pensanti's Cream: Helen Pensanti, MD, Inc., P.O. Box 7530, Newport Beach, CA 92658, (714) 542-8333, fax: (949) 856-4573, e-mail: info@askdrhelen.com and orders@askdrhelen.com, www.askdrhelen.com.

Dr. Randolph's Natural Progesterone Cream, toll-free (866) 628-6337, www.womens-medicine.com. This is Dr. Randy Randolph's cream, which contains only progesterone as its active ingredient and no chemicals.

Easy Way International, 4610 Arrowhead Drive, Carson City, NV 89706, (800) 267-4522. They make Gentle Changes progesterone cream.

Emerita, a division of Transitions for Health, Inc., 621 SW Alder, Suite 900, Portland, OR 97205-3627, (503) 226-1010 or (800) 648-8211. Pro-Gest is the original natural progesterone cream.

Goldshield Elite, 1501 Northpoint Parkway, Suite 100, West Palm Beach, FL 22407, (866) 218-8142. (They have operators for English, French and Spanish speakers, and distribution in Europe, Canada, and the United States), e-mail: cs@goldshieldelite.com, www.goldshieldelite.com. Rejuvenate Crème.

The Health and Science Research Institute, 1648 Taylor Road, Suite 118, Port Orange, FL 32128, (888) 222-1415, fax: (904) 756-0194, www.health-science.com. Serenity for Women progesterone cream, which contains no petrochemical products.

HM Enterprises, 2622 Bailey Drive, Norcross, GA 30071, (800) 742-4773, e-mail: proge@hmenterprises.com, www .hmenterprises.com or www.paulbunyan.net/users/mlzeller. They make Happy PMS progesterone cream.

International Health, 2401 N. Hayden Road, Scottsdale, AZ 85257, toll-free (800) 481-9987 or (480) 874-1419, www.ihsite.com, e-mail: nopms@doitnow.com. Makers of EssPro'Leve Plus Progesterone Cream with Essential Oils.

Kevala, a division of Karuna, 42 Digital Drive #7, Novato, CA 94949, (888) 749-8643, e-mail: info@kevalahealth .com, www.kevalahealth.com. They make PureGest Lotion, which is free from additional hormones, herbs, and alcohols.

Kokoro, LLC., P.O. Box 597, Tustin, CA 92781, (800) 599-9412, (714) 836-7749, www.kokorohealth.com. They offer Kokoro Women's Balance Crème.

Life Extension, P.O. Box 229120, Hollywood, FL 33022, (800) 544-4440, (954) 766-8433, e-mail: customerservice @lifeextension.com, www.lifeextension.com. Makers of Pro-Fem Cream.

Life-flo Health Care Products, 8146 N. 23rd Avenue, Suite E, Phoenix, AZ 85021, (888) 999-7440, e-mail: care@life-flo.com, www.life-flo.com or www.sheld.com/ lifeflo/. They make Progestacare cream.

Natural Pause-Natural Menopause Solutions, 8665 W. Flamingo Road, Suite 131-413, Las Vegas, NV 89147, (888) 267-5032, e-mail: info@naturalpause.com, www .naturalpause.com. Makers of Natural Pause cream.

Products of Nature, 54 Danbury Road, Ridgefield, CT 06877, (800) 665-5952. www.pronature.com, www .prodnature.com. Maker of Natural Woman progesterone cream.

Sarati International, Rt. 3, Box 385, Ted Hunt Road, Los Fresno, TX 78566, (800) 900-0701, www.sarati.com. On-line distributors: www.sunrisewd.com or www.progestnet .com. They make Natural Progesterone Cream.

Springboard, 3115 Stoney Oak Drive, Spring Valley, CA 91978, toll-free (866) 882-6868, or (619) 670-3860, fax: (619) 670-4149, www.springboard4health.com or www.naturalprogesterone.com. They make ProBalance progesterone cream.

Vitamin Research Products, Inc., 4610 Arrowhead Drive. Carson City, NV 89706, (775) 884-1300, (800) 877-2447, www.vrp.com. Makers of HerBalance Cream.

Women's Health America, Inc., 1289 Deming Way, Madison, WI 53717, (800) 558-7046, e-mail: wha@womenshealth .com, www.womenshealth.com. Restore BioBalance Progesterone Cream.

Zand, 1441 West Smith Road, Ferndale, WA 98248, (800) 232-4005, fax: (360) 384-1140, www.zand.com, www .drugstore.com. Progesterone Menopause Cream, fragrance free, no petrochemicals.

Compounding Pharmacists

www.iacprx.org. If your doctor is interested in natural hormones but hesitant about prescribing an over-the-counter cream, you can put him/her in touch with a compounding pharmacist skilled in the use of natural hormone supplements, who can educate your physician and provide dosing guidelines. For a referral in your area contact IACP (International Academy of Compounding

Pharmacists), (800) 927-4227, ext. 300, or go online to the website address above.

Progesterone Cream in the United Kingdom

Institute of Well-Being, P.O. Box 493, St. Peter Port, Guernsey, GY1 6BY, UK, 01481 258225, e-mail: sales@pro-gest.co.uk, www.pro-gest.co.uk. Emerita's Pro-Gest cream, available tax-free and no prescription required.

References

For a complete list of references, please refer to our other books, listed below.

Other Warner Books by John R. Lee, M.D., and Virginia Hopkins

What Your Doctor May Not Tell You About Menopause: The Breakthrough Book on Natural Progesterone (Warner Books, 1996).

What Your Doctor May Not Tell You About Premenopause: Balance Your Hormones and Your Life from Thirty to Fifty (Warner Books, 1999).

What Your Doctor May Not Tell You About Breast Cancer: How Hormone Balance Can Help Save Your Life (Warner Books, 2002).

Index

Index

food. *See* diet
food labels, 170
formaldehyde, 168
fragrances, 168, 169–72
Framingham Study, 151

gallbladder pain, 47, 76
glucose. *See* blood sugar
grapefruit juice, 89–90

hair, dry and brittle, 45
hair loss, 47, 76, 93
hands, cold, 44
headaches, 47, 49, 76, 102
heart disease, 59–60, 98
heart palpitations, 48
Heparin, 160
Hopkins, Virginia, 4, 7
Hormone Balance for Men (Lee), 7–8
Hormone Balance Test, 28–34
  symptom group 1 (progesterone
    deficiency), 29, 32
  symptom group 2 (estrogen
    deficiency), 30, 32
  symptom group 3 (estrogen
    excess), 30, 32–33
  symptom group 4 (estrogen
    dominance), 31, 33
  symptom group 5 (androgen
    excess), 31, 33
  symptom group 6 (cortisol
    deficiency), 31, 33–34
hormone basics, 9–14
hormone cycles, 13–14
hormone level tests, 55–58. *See
  also* blood tests; saliva tests
hormone replacement therapy
  (HRT), 15–16, 59–60, 63–72
  defined, 10
  Three Rules for, 18–26, 175
hot flashes, 48, 64, 77, 123

hyperglycemia, 159–60
hypoglycemia, 48, 77, 102
hysterectomy, 88, 91, 94, 119, 124

incontinence, 48, 92
insomnia, 48–49, 77
insulin, 148–50, 157–60
insulin resistance, 151–52, 157–59
intercourse, painful, 51, 77
irregular bleeding, 140–41
irritability, 49, 77, 93, 102
irritable bowel syndrome, 73

journal, for recording lifestyle,
  40–41

Lee, John R.
  life and work of, 1–8
  Three Rules for HRT, 18–26, 175
Leonetti, Helen, 70
leptin, 166
lethargy, 52, 111
libido (sex drive), 44, 76, 92,
  93–94, 112
lifestyle choices, 27, 37, 145–46.
  See also diet; exercise; stress
  journal for recording, 40–41
loading dose, 127–29
low-carb diets, 147–48, 152–54
luteal insufficiency, 126–27

medroxyprogesterone acetate. *See*
  Provera
Megace, 13
memory loss, 49, 77, 165
men, hormone balance for, 7–8
Menest, 66
menopause, 118–19, 123, 136,
  137–39
  defined, 14
  insulin resistance and, 158–59

About the Authors

JOHN R. LEE, M.D., (1929–2003) was internationally acknowledged as a pioneer and expert in the study and use of the hormone progesterone, and on the subject of hormone replacement therapy for women. He used transdermal progesterone extensively in his clinical practice for nearly a decade, doing research that showed it can reverse osteoporosis. Dr. Lee also famously coined the term "estrogen dominance," meaning a relative lack of progesterone compared to estrogen, which causes a list of symptoms familiar to millions of women. Dr. Lee had a distinguished medical career, including graduating from Harvard and the University of Minnesota Medical School. After he retired from a 30-year family practice in northern California, he began writing and traveling around the world speaking to doctors, scientists, and lay people about progesterone. Dr. Lee also taught a very popular course on "Optimal Health" at the College of Marin for 15 years, for which he wrote the book *Optimal Health Guidelines*. His second self-published book, written for doctors, was *Natural Progesterone: The Multiple Roles of a Remarkable Hormone*. He then teamed up with Virginia Hopkins and others to write the best sellers *What Your Doctor May Not Tell You About Menopause* and *What Your Doctor May Not Tell You About Premenopause,* as well as *What Your Doctor May Not Tell You About Breast Cancer.*

Virginia Hopkins, M.A., has been a writer and editor since she graduated from Yale University in 1976. She has a master's degree in Applied Psychology from the University of Santa Monica. She is the co-author, with John R. Lee, M.D., of *What Your Doctor May Not Tell You About Menopause* (Warner Books, 1996, 2003), *What Your Doctor May Not Tell You About Premenopause* (Warner Books, 1999), *What Your Doctor May Not Tell You About Breast Cancer* (Warner Books, 2002), and she co-authored *Prescription Alternatives* (Keats Publishing, 1998), with Earl Mindell, R.Ph., Ph.D. She writes the e-mail newsletter "The Hopkins Health Watch" (www.hopkinshealthwatch.com), has a website that sells test kits (www.hopkinstestkits.com), and has written or co-authored more than 35 books on alternative health and nutrition.